Understandi

DIABE

GW00320098

Dr Rudy Bilous

Published by Family Doctor Publications Limited
in association with the British Medical Association

IMPORTANT NOTICE

This book is not designed as a substitute for personal medical advice
but as a supplement to that advice for the patient who wishes to
understand more about his/her condition.

Before taking any form of treatment YOU SHOULD ALWAYS
CONSULT YOUR MEDICAL PRACTITIONER

In particular (without limit) you should note that advances in medical
science occur rapidly and some of the information contained in this
booklet about drugs and treatment may very soon be out of date.

THIS IS THE 1998 EDITION

First edition 1995
Reprinted 1996, 1998

With contributions from Lorna Hall, BSc and Debbie Black, BSc, Senior Dietitians, South
Tees Acute Hospitals Trust, and Sharon Martin, Chief IV Chiropodist, South Tees
Community and Mental Health Trust

Family Doctor Publications, 10 Butchers Row, Banbury, Oxon OX16 8JH

Medical Editor: Dr Tony Smith
Consultant Editor: Chris McLaughlin
Cover Artist: Dave Eastbury
Illustrator: Angela Christie
Design: MPG Design, Blandford Forum, Dorset
Printing: Reflex Litho, Thetford, Norfolk, using acid-free paper

ISBN: 1-898205-10-8

visit.our.web.site
www.familydoctor.co.uk

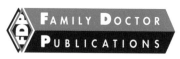 **FAMILY DOCTOR PUBLICATIONS** Welcome!

Family Doctor books

...backing up your doctor's consultation

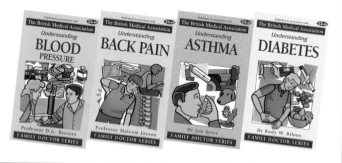

---

home
– general information

news
of new titles

books
– details and extracts

useful links
to other organisations

audio cassettes
for self help

contact us
with your enquiries

Contents

Introduction 1

Making a diagnosis 7

Treatment: diet 10

Treatment: medication 20

Checking your glucose levels 30

All about hypoglycaemia 36

Breaking your routine 42

Children with diabetes 50

If it gets complicated 54

Who cares? 65

Questions & answers 68

Future prospects for people with diabetes 71

Useful addresses 74

Index 75

Introduction

If you have just found out that you have diabetes, this doesn't mean that you have become sick or turned into an invalid. Millions of people in this country have diabetes and most lead normal, active lives. Some of them have had the condition for over 50 years. With advances in our understanding of the disease and improvements in treatment, the prospects for someone with diabetes are better than ever before. This book is meant to help you understand what diabetes is and how to control it. Doctors nowadays encourage people with diabetes to take a lot of responsibility for their own health, paying careful attention to their diet and carrying out regular tests on their blood and urine to monitor their progress. We shall explain, step by step, how you can do this and develop confidence that you really are in control of your diabetes.

Diabetes is one of the oldest known human diseases. Its full name – diabetes mellitus – comes from the Greek words for syphon and sugar and describes the most obvious symptom of uncontrolled diabetes: the passing of large amounts of urine which is sweet because it contains sugar (glucose). There are descriptions of the symptoms by the ancient Persians, Indians and Egyptians, but a proper understanding of the condition has only developed over the last hundred years or so.

In the later part of the nineteenth century, two German doctors worked out that the pancreas – a large gland behind the stomach – must be producing some substance which stopped the level of blood glucose rising. In 1921 three Canadian scientists discovered that the mystery substance, which they named insulin, was produced in small groups of cells within the pancreas called the islets of Langerhans. When insulin became available as a treatment for diabetes after 1922, it was seen as a medical miracle, transforming the future prospects of sufferers and saving the lives of many young people who would otherwise have died after a painful wasting illness. Some

regular injections of insulin to remain well.

● **Non-insulin-dependent diabetes mellitus (NIDDM):** Also called type 2, age-related or maturity onset, this is more common in middle or later life and can be controlled by tablets or just by diet.

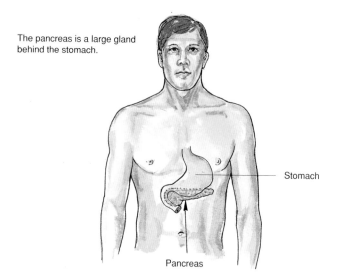

The pancreas is a large gland behind the stomach.

Stomach

Pancreas

30 years later, it was found that one form of diabetes could be treated with tablets to lower levels of blood glucose. This new development led doctors to distinguish between two forms of the condition.

● **Insulin-dependent diabetes mellitus (IDDM):** Also called type 1, this starts most commonly in younger patients who have to have

WHAT IS DIABETES?

It is a permanent change in your internal chemistry which results in you having too much glucose in your blood. The cause is a deficiency of the hormone insulin. A hormone is a chemical messenger that is made in one part of the body (in this case the pancreas) and is released into the bloodstream to have an effect on more distant parts. There may be complete failure of insulin production as in type 1. In type 2, however, there is usually a combination of a partial failure of insulin production, and a reduced body response to the hormone. This is called insulin resistance.

WHAT GOES WRONG?

The glucose in your blood comes from the digestion of food and the chemical changes made to it by the liver. Some glucose is stored and some is used for energy. Insulin has a unique shape that plugs into special sockets or receptors on the surface of cells throughout the body. By plugging into these receptors, insulin makes cells extract glucose from the blood and also prevents them from breaking down proteins and fat. It is the only hormone that can reduce blood glucose, and does this in several ways:

- By increasing the amount stored in the liver in the form of glycogen
- By preventing the liver from releasing too much glucose
- By encouraging cells elsewhere in the body to take up glucose.

Other mechanisms in the body work in conjunction with insulin to help maintain the correct level of blood glucose. However, insulin is the only means the body has of actually lowering blood glucose levels, so when the insulin supply fails, the whole system goes out of balance. After a meal, there is no brake on the glucose absorbed from what you've eaten, so the level in your blood goes on rising. When the concentration rises above a certain level, the glucose starts to spill out of the bloodstream into the urine. Infections such as cystitis and thrush can develop more easily when the urine is sweet as the germs responsible can grow more rapidly.

Another consequence of rising blood glucose is a tendency to pass more urine. This is because the extra glucose in the blood is filtered out by the kidneys which try to dispose of it by excreting more salt and water. This excess urine production is called polyuria and is often the earliest sign of diabetes. If nothing is done to halt this process, the person will quickly become dehydrated and thirsty. As previously mentioned, as well as regulating blood glucose, insulin acts to prevent weight loss and help build up body tissue – so a person whose supply has failed or isn't working properly will inevitably lose some weight.

SYMPTOMS

The severity of the symptoms and the rate at which they develop may

- Thirst
- Dehydration
- Passing large quantities of urine
- Urinary tract infection (such as cystitis) or thrush
- Weight loss
- Tiredness and lethargy
- Blurred vision resulting from dehydration of the lens in the eye

differ depending on which type of diabetes you have.

Type 1 (IDDM)

As the person isn't producing any insulin at all, the symptoms can come on very rapidly as blood glucose control is lost. Insulin has a very important role in maintaining stability in the body by preventing breakdown of proteins (found in muscle) and fats. When insulin fails, the by-products of the breakdown of fat and muscle build up in the blood and lead to the production of substances called ketones. If nothing is done to stop this, the level will rise until eventually it causes the person to go into what's called a ketoacidotic coma. This is much less common these days as diabetes is usually diagnosed long before coma develops. However, when it occurs patients need urgent hospital treatment with insulin and fluids into a vein. This is not the same thing as a coma induced by low blood sugar (or hypoglycaemia) – see page 36.

Type 2 (NIDDM)

As the supply of insulin is reduced or is not quite as effective as normal, the blood glucose level rises more slowly. There is less protein and fat breakdown so ketones are produced in much smaller quantities and the risk of a ketoacidotic coma is low.

WHO GETS IT?

Around two per cent of people in this country have diabetes, although as many as half of them may not realise it. The vast majority have type 2, and more women than men are affected, probably because diabetes is more common later in life and women tend to live longer. As the age of the population as a whole is rising, type 2 diabetes is likely to become even more common over the coming years.

There are several known reasons why insulin secretion may be reduced, and any individual could be affected by one or more of them.

Genetic

Researchers studying identical twins and the family trees of patients with diabetes have found that heredity is an important factor in both kinds of diabetes. With type 1 diabetes, there is about a 50 per cent chance of the second twin developing the condition if the first one has it, and a five per cent chance of the child of an affected parent doing so. With type 2 diabetes, it is virtually certain that, if one of a pair of identical twins develops it, the other will do so as well.

It is difficult to predict precisely who will inherit the condition. A small number of families have a much stronger tendency to develop diabetes and scientists have identified several genes which seem to be involved. In these circumstances, it may be possible to test family members and determine their risk of developing the condition.

For the most part, however, it is difficult to identify the genes involved and this makes it different from some other conditions such as cystic fibrosis, where a single gene is operating. So even if a close member of your family has diabetes, there is no certainty that you will develop it yourself. Some people who inherit a tendency to diabetes never actually get it, so there are obviously other factors at work here.

Infection

It has been known for some time that type 1 in children and young people is more likely to come on at certain times of the year when there are a lot of coughs and colds about. Some viruses, such as mumps and Coxsackie, are known to have the potential to damage the pancreas, bringing on diabetes. As far as individual patients are concerned, however, it is very rare that doctors can link the onset of their diabetes with a specific bout of infection. A possible explanation for this is that the infection may have begun a process which only comes to light many years later.

Environmental

People who develop type 2 are often overweight and eat an unbalanced diet. It's interesting to note that people who move from a country with a low risk to one where there's a higher risk have the same chance of developing diabetes as the locals in their new country. Dramatic changes in lifestyle, too, can make it more likely that a person will get diabetes.

A good example of this is shown by the Pacific islanders of Nauru who became very wealthy when phosphates were discovered on their island. As a consequence, their diets changed dramatically and they put on a lot of weight and became much more prone to developing diabetes.

All this points to important connections between diet, environment and diabetes. However, there is not a precise link between developing diabetes and the individual consumption of sugar and sweets.

Secondary diabetes

There are a small number of people who develop diabetes as a result of other disease of the pancreas. For example, pancreatitis (or inflammation of the pancreas) can bring on the condition by destroying large parts of the gland. Some people suffering from hormonal diseases, such as Cushing's syndrome (the body makes too much steroid hormone) or acromegaly (the body makes too much growth hormone), may also have diabetes as a side effect of their main illness. It can also be a result of damage to the pancreas caused by chronic over-indulgence in alcohol.

Stress

Although many people relate the onset of their diabetes to a stressful event such as an accident or other illness, it is difficult to prove a direct link between stress and diabetes. The explanation may lie in the fact that people see their doctors because of some stressful event, and their diabetes is diagnosed opportunistically at the same time.

KEY POINTS

✓ Diabetes arises when an individual cannot make enough insulin or the insulin that he or she does make is ineffective at controlling blood glucose levels

✓ Insulin is a hormone (chemical messenger) that is critical for maintaining healthy life

✓ Symptoms of diabetes are weight loss, passing more urine, thirst and feeling run down

✓ There are several causes including genetic (inherited) predisposition, infections, environmental factors and stress, and any or all of these may be important in each individual case

Making a diagnosis

People find out they have the condition in different ways.

With type 2, the first port of call is usually your GP, either because you have some or all of the symptoms listed on page 4, or because you are having a general check-up. Some people are advised to see their doctor by their optician. This is because an eye examination will pick up the early signs of a condition called diabetic retinopathy – changes in the blood vessels of the eye which can develop as a complication of diabetes (see page 57).

If your symptoms suggest to your doctor that you may have diabetes, he will want to do a blood test to measure your glucose level, and will also ask for a urine sample to be tested. The samples may have to be sent off to the lab for analysis, although many GPs today have blood glucose meters in the surgery, and can give you the result on the spot.

Above-average readings from either or both of these tests will probably be sufficient for your doctor to confirm that you have diabetes and, if it's type 2, it's likely that you will be cared for by your GP rather than having to see a hospital doctor. Many GP practices run regular diabetes clinics, but if yours doesn't or you feel you need more support, you can ask to be referred to a hospital diabetes clinic.

As mentioned above, type 1 can often come on quite suddenly, and this may mean the person being admitted to hospital while the diagnosis is made and the condition stabilised. People with this form of diabetes will probably continue to be under the care of the specialist team at a hospital.

Nowadays, many type 1 and type 2 patients have shared care

between the hospital and the GP.

Although, for most people, the diagnosis is straightforward and quite clear cut, a few may need an extra test because their blood glucose level is borderline. In this case, you may be asked to go to the hospital outpatients clinic for what's called an oral glucose tolerance test. After an overnight fast, your blood glucose level will be measured on arrival, then you'll be given a drink containing a measured amount of glucose. Your blood will then be retested at half-hourly intervals for two hours to see how your body is dealing with the glucose you've absorbed. You may also be asked to pass a urine sample at the start and at hourly intervals.

ORAL GLUCOSE TOLERANCE TEST

There are three possible outcomes, depending on the results of your test:

- Your blood glucose may be within the normal range, so you don't have diabetes.

- Your level may be higher than average, although not high enough to mean you have diabetes. This condition is called impaired glucose tolerance (IGT) and your medical advisers will want to keep an eye on you because there is a possibility of developing diabetes in the future. In the meantime you will be given advice on diet, although you don't have diabetes and don't need any other specific treatment.

- Your blood glucose level may be sufficiently raised to indicate that you do have diabetes. If so, you will need to see your doctor to discuss what treatment you need.

KEY POINTS

✓ Diabetes is usually diagnosed from a simple urine or blood test in patients who have symptoms (see page 4)

✓ A small number of patients need to have a more formal test called an oral glucose tolerance test

✓ Early diagnosis is very important and patients with symptoms are recommended to attend their GP's surgery for a test

Treatment: diet

Diabetes can be tackled in three main ways.

Diet

A diabetic diet actually means following a healthy eating plan rather than a difficult or restrictive programme. This applies to everyone with diabetes, regardless of which type they have, and may be enough by itself to control type 2 in some people. However, if you have type 1, you will need to learn about balancing your intake of food with your insulin injections in order to achieve the best possible control of your blood glucose levels.

Tablets

These are used to control type 2 and there are different types. For more about this kind of treatment, see page 20.

Insulin

Everyone with type 1 will have to take insulin by injection, but only a minority of those with type 2 will be treated this way. More about insulin on page 22.

YOUR HEALTHY EATING PLAN

The sort of diet you should follow when you have diabetes definitely does not mean a future of self-denial on the food front. What it does mean is eating more of the foods that are good for you, and cutting right down on those that are not so good, but actually it's the kind of eating which experts recommend for everyone, whether they have diabetes or not. The difference it can make to your overall health and well-being is even more worthwhile when you

WHAT SHOULD YOU WEIGH?

- The body mass index (BMI) is a useful measure of healthy weight
- Find out your height in metres and weight in kilograms
- Calculate your BMI like this:

$$BMI = \frac{\text{Your weight (kg)}}{[\text{Your height (metres)} \times \text{your height (metres)}]}$$

e.g. $24.8 = \dfrac{70}{[1.68 \times 1.68]}$

(handwritten) (2014) $\dfrac{79}{1.68^2} = 28$

(handwritten) 2014 (28) 2015 (26)

- You are recommended to try to maintain a BMI in the range 20–25
- The chart below is an easier way of estimating your BMI. Read off your height and your weight. Where the lines cross in the chart indicates your range of BMI

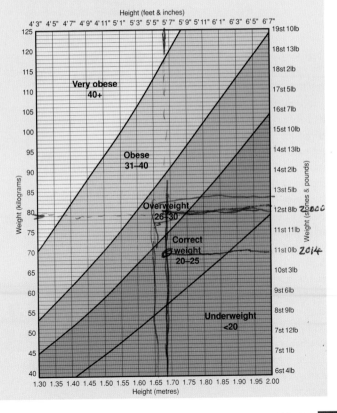

✓ • Cut down on fried and fatty foods (see 'Fat – who needs it?' on page 16)

✓ • Eat smaller portions

✓ • Cut out snacks such as crisps and biscuits; try fruit instead ?

✓ • Eat regular meals

? • Take more exercise

do have diabetes, however, because without it your medication will not be nearly as effective.

Regular meals

The other thing to remember is that you'll find it easier to keep your blood glucose under control if you stick to regular mealtimes. If you're on insulin, your dietitian or nurse will explain about the importance of dovetailing meals with injections, and you'll gradually work out your own way of matching your food intake to your energy output. This may be particularly difficult at first for those who work shifts. Your diabetes care team or your GP will advise you, but basically you should aim to have a substantial meal or a snack every three to four hours and work your medication around this schedule.

You may need extra meals or snacks at night when you're actually working.

? High Sugar Try Shredded Wheat

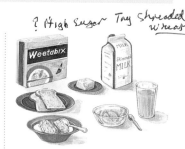

Breakfast

3%

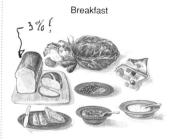

Main meal

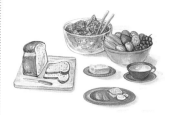

Snack meal

HEALTHY EATING MENU – BREAKFAST

- Skimmed or semi-skimmed milk ← Soya < 0.5% ✓   *(handwritten: 3%)*
- Artificial sweetener instead of sugar ✓
- High-fibre cereal, e.g. porridge, Branflakes, Weetabix, Shredded Wheat ✓
- Wholemeal or wholegrain bread ✓
- Poly- or monounsaturated or low-fat spreads ✓
- Low-sugar jam or marmalade ✓
- Fruit ✓ ?   *(handwritten: Bananas ✗, very ripe fruits ✗)*

MAIN MEAL

- Include some starchy food – bread, potatoes, pasta, rice or chapatti, for example ✓
- At least two portions of vegetables, and try to include peas and <u>beans</u> as often as possible ✓
- Small portions of lean meat or fish. Cut off fat, and avoid frying ✓ *(handwritten: oil/fat free grilling ✓)*
- Fresh or tinned fruit (in natural, unsweetened juices), plus unsweetened/sugar-free jelly or custard .
- Diet/virtually fat-free or natural yoghurts

SNACK MEALS

- Bread, pasta, chapatti or jacket potatoes – go for low-fat fillings such as lean meat, <u>baked beans</u>, low-fat cheese or tinned fish (not in oil) ✓ *(handwritten: ✗ Sugar 30%)*
- Fresh or tinned fruit in natural juice ✗
- Vegetables or salad ✓

BETWEEN MEALS – SNACKS/SUPPER

- Avoid eating too many of these if you're trying to lose weight, and stick to fruit instead
- Sandwiches or toast with low-fat fillings
- Bowl of cereal or porridge
- Low-fat crisps
- Plain biscuits
- Toasted crumpets and muffins

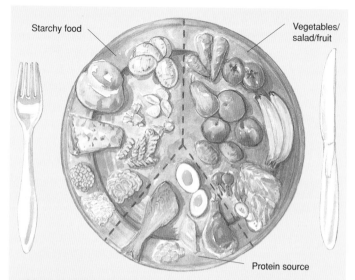

Starchy food

Vegetables/salad/fruit

Protein source

At each meal your food contribution needs to be in the above illustrated proportions.

Two-fifths of your plate should be covered with starchy food preferably of high-fibre variety. *Keep low*

Two-fifths of your plate should be covered with vegetables/salad or fruit. ✓

The remaining one-fifth of your plate should be a protein source, for example, meat, fish, eggs, pulses or cheese. ✓

By ensuring that these proportions of nutrient sources are achieved and maintained, your blood glucose should stay within desirable ranges.

Controlling your weight

People whose diabetes is newly diagnosed may well be advised to lose some weight – if you're not sure, check the chart on page 11.

Once your new eating plan is established, you'll probably find that it's easy to maintain a stable weight, but in the meantime, it's worth following a few simple guidelines.

Remember that you will only lose weight if you eat less food than your body needs to carry out its daily activities. The headings on the following pages can be used as guidelines to a healthier way of eating. There's no reason why everyone in the family shouldn't enjoy the benefits of your 'diabetic' diet but, if some of them are big fans of fried food or sweet puddings, you may find it better to introduce the changes gradually rather than all at once.

Often you'll find that you can eat a meal which tastes very much like what you're used to, but is better for you because it includes the healthier versions of familiar foods. Our healthy eating menu (see page 13) shows how you might do this, substituting the foods listed for your usual ones.

A BALANCED DIET

As you'll realise by now, healthy eating means having a good mix of the right kind of food, and cutting back on those which can do more harm than good. If you really are confused or worried about what you should be eating, ask to see a dietitian who can put you straight. Once you get used to the basics, however, it's mostly quite simple, as you will see from our guidelines on the next few pages.

Carbohydrates

These foods are broken down in your body to produce glucose, which gives you energy. There are two types: sugary and starchy.

• **Sugary**: Sugar, sweets and choco-

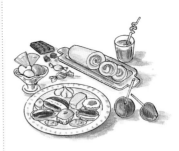

Sugary

late, cakes, sweet biscuits and puddings, fizzy drinks, for example. You have to steer clear of these because the glucose gets into your bloodstream very fast, and can cause a sudden rise in your blood glucose level.

You can use artificial sweeteners such as saccharine, aspartame and acesulfame, on cereals and in drinks instead of sugar. It's OK to use a small amount of ordinary sugar for baking cakes, but keep these for main meals – and don't forget the calorie content!

• **Starchy**: Bread, potatoes, pasta, rice, cereals and fruit, for example. These are slower acting and are

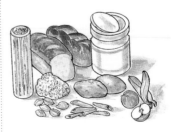

Starchy

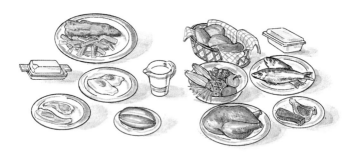

Cut down on these   Choose these instead

good sources of energy, so eat them regularly throughout the day, and try to include some at each meal time.

Fat – who needs it?

The type of fat that we eat is also important. There are two main types: saturated and unsaturated.

- **Saturated (animal) fat**: Found in fatty meats, full-cream milk, butter and lard, for example, this type can cause problems for the circulation (see 'If it gets complicated' on page 54). Everyone needs to reduce their intake of this kind of fat.

- **Unsaturated fats**: These are slightly better than saturated fats and come in two forms.

Polyunsaturated fats are found in sunflower oil, pure vegetable oil, corn oil and sunflower margarines, for example.

Monounsaturated fats are found in olive oil, rape seed oil and

safflower oil, for example. This type of fat should be used instead of saturated and polyunsaturated fat whenever possible.

Remember that all fats are high in calories and so will lead to weight gain if taken in excess.

Fibre

Fibre (also called roughage) can be either soluble (dissolves in water and slows absorption of food) or insoluble (cannot be digested and helps to prevent constipation). Insoluble fibre is also useful when you are slimming because it makes you feel full up.

Increasing the fibre content of your diet doesn't mean having brown rice and bran with every-thing, but you should aim to consume around 30 grams of fibre a day. It is essential to keep your intestine working well, and some types such as soluble fibre can help with both good blood glucose control and keeping your blood cholesterol levels down. Foods such as baked beans, mushy peas, lentil soup and dahl, plus oat-based dishes like porridge and other cereals and oat cakes, are high in soluble fibre. Food such as high-fibre cereals, wholemeal or granary bread, unpeeled vegetables and fruit, plus wholemeal versions of pasta, flour and rice have mainly insoluble fibre.

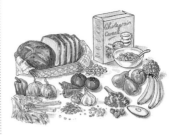

Increase your intake of fibre

Proteins

These are necessary so your body can repair tissue and to fuel normal growth in children – but you don't need that much, and probably less than you think. Aim to have about

ALCOHOL

Having diabetes doesn't mean turning teetotal unless you prefer to, but you do have to follow a few commonsense rules, particularly if you are on tablets or insulin. Remember that alcohol can cause hypoglycaemia (low blood glucose, see page 36).

- Limit yourself to three 'units' or less in any one day. One unit of alcohol means a single measure of spirits, half a pint of beer or a small glass of wine.

- Avoid 'diabetic' or Pils-type beers or lagers because, although they have less sugar, they are high in alcohol and more likely to cause a low blood glucose.

- Make sure you eat a meal containing carbohydrates whenever you drink alcohol.

- You may find that your face flushes red if you mix alcohol with some kinds of tablet treatment.

- Remember to allow for the calorie content of alcoholic drinks and mixers, which should be diet/slimline versions.

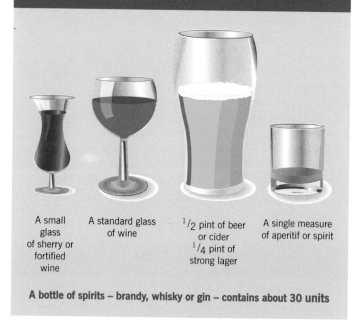

A UNIT OF ALCOHOL IS

A small glass of sherry or fortified wine

A standard glass of wine

$^1/_2$ pint of beer or cider
$^1/_4$ pint of strong lager

A single measure of aperitif or spirit

A bottle of spirits – brandy, whisky or gin – contains about 30 units

12 to 15 per cent of your daily energy requirements in the form of protein. This can come either from cereal sources (bread, cereals, rice, pasta, flour) or animal sources (meat, fish, eggs and dairy produce). Animal proteins tend to be relatively high in fats and calories and contain no carbohydrates, so this needs to be taken into account when planning your diet.

Salt

Too much salt is not good for us and can lead to high blood pressure. Try to use a small amount in cooking and don't add any more at the table. Herbs, spices and pepper can be used to add more flavour to your food as necessary.

Vitamins and minerals

If you're eating a well-balanced diet, you really shouldn't need to take any vitamin or mineral supplements. Some researchers have suggested that deficiencies of elements such as chromium and selenium may have a role in the onset of diabetic complications. However, the problem is that there is no way of measuring either the quantities in your diet or the levels present in your body. So your best bet is probably to eat as varied a diet as possible to ensure that you get enough of these elements along with all the other nutrients.

KEY POINTS

✓ Eat regularly

✓ Include some starchy food (carbohydrate) with each meal, choosing high-fibre versions where possible

✓ Reduce your fat intake and remember to watch the type of fat

✓ Limit your intake of sugars and sugary foods

✓ Aim to keep to your ideal body weight and exercise regularly when possible

✓ Use salt sparingly

✓ Do not drink too much alcohol

Treatment: medication

WHEN YOU'RE ON TABLETS

There are four main kinds of tablet treatment for people with type 2 diabetes: (1) sulphonylureas, (2) biguanides, (3) acarbose and (4) thiazolidinediones. They all come under the general name of oral hypoglycaemic agents (OHAs), and any of them may be taken alone or in combination. Most people with type 2 find that these medications, together with a healthy eating pattern, keep their diabetes well under control, although it may take a while to find out which combination or dose suits you best. If you do experience side effects or find that your blood glucose levels are higher than they should be, you should go back to your GP to discuss possible changes to your treatment.

Sulphonylureas (SUs)

These work by stimulating the pancreas to release stored insulin. You could say that they raise your insulin level by proxy, and so help to keep blood glucose down. You have to remember that, although you're not actually taking insulin, these tablets have a similar effect because they increase the amount of insulin in your bloodstream, and it is possible for it to increase too much. If this happens, your blood glucose levels will drop too far, and you may sometimes experience the symptoms of hypoglycaemia (see page 36). To prevent this happening, you should make sure you eat regularly, and take your tablets either with or just before a meal.

As with insulin, SUs can be short, medium or long acting (see below), and must be taken once, twice or three times a day depending on how fast they work. The long-acting versions do not always suit older people or those whose lifestyle makes it difficult to have regular meal times because of the risk of hypoglycaemia.

Apart from having to be aware

NAMES OF SULPHONYLUREA TABLETS AVAILABLE IN THE UK

Chemical name	Trade name	Duration of action
Chlorpropamide	Diabinese	Long
Glibenclamide	Daonil/Euglucon	Medium
Gliclazide	Diamicron	Medium
Glipizide	Glibenese/Minodiab	Medium
Gliquidone	Glurenorm	Medium
Tolazamide	Tolanase	Medium
Tolbutamide	Rastinon	Short

of the risk of low blood glucose, most people taking SUs find they have few if any serious side effects. Probably the most annoying one is that most patients find that their face can get very flushed and hot when they drink alcohol. The precise reasons for this side effect are unclear. As you'll soon discover once you're taking them, the fact that SUs lower your blood glucose will make you feel very hungry so you could gain a lot of weight if you're not careful.

A minority of people won't be able to take SUs because they're allergic to them, and if you're allergic to the antibiotic Septrin you may also have a reaction to SUs.

Biguanides

This type of drug has been in use for over 50 years, and the only one available in this country is metformin. No one is sure precisely how it works, but it seems to slow down the absorption of glucose from the intestines and may also have a more complicated effect on the liver. As a result of this, you can't take it if you have any kind of liver disease, and it is also best avoided in patients with kidney complications (see page 58). You don't have to worry about your blood glucose level dropping too far when you're on metformin because it doesn't stimulate the release of insulin. It's often pre-scribed for people who are over-weight because it doesn't make you feel hungry or put on extra pounds. You normally start on a low dose, taking it once or twice a day with meals, and then gradually build up the amount you're taking as you get used to it.

The main side effects are

stomach upsets – nausea and diarrhoea – and some people have to stop taking it because of this problem.

Acarbose

This works in quite a different way from the other OHAs. By interfering with the breakdown of carbo-hydrates into sugar, it stops your body from absorbing glucose from food.

Unfortunately, this means that more sugars remain unabsorbed in the large intestine where lots of bacteria and micro-organisms lurk. These feed on the abundant sugar and proliferate, which can mean you suffer from loose motions and flatus. Nevertheless, it could be the right option for you if you find it difficult to follow a healthy eating plan or tend to be overweight.

Thiazolidinediones

This new class of drugs improves sensitivity to insulin and thus enables the hormone to lower blood glucose more effectively. The first drug in this group, troglitazone, has been shown to be very effective but has been withdrawn temporarily because of side effects in the liver. More examples of these drugs will become available in the near future. As these tablets also do not stimulate insulin release, hypo-glycaemia (low blood glucose) and weight gain are not a problem.

WHEN YOU NEED INSULIN

When you have type 1 diabetes, there's no alternative to replacing the missing insulin by means of daily injections. A proportion of people whose type 2 diabetes is not effectively controlled by diet and tablets may also have to change to a regimen of insulin injections. If you've just found this out, it's bound to take you a while to adjust to the idea but with the right information and back-up from your diabetes care team, you'll soon realise that you will be able to cope and keep yourself well. They will show you how to give injections, and take time to teach you how to manage your condition effectively. Don't worry if you need to see them several times to get things clear – no one will mind. In fact, they will encourage you to keep asking questions and coming back until you feel comfortable with all the masses of new information. Here we will look at some of the questions people with newly diagnosed diabetes ask most often.

Why do I have to inject the insulin?

This is the only effective way of getting it into your bloodstream. If you swallow it, it is partly digested and so becomes less active, which means it can't do its job of con-trolling your blood glucose level. Although other ways of giving insulin have been tried, they've all had problems, so injection is the only practical option for the time being.

Why is insulin injected under the skin?

In theory, it could be injected into a vein or a muscle, as happens with some other medicines such as antibiotics. In practice, however, injecting the insulin into a vein several times a day would be difficult, and intramuscular injections can be painful. Both these methods are sometimes used in special circumstances – for instance, when you are ill or can't eat regularly, perhaps because you're having an operation.

What types of insulin are there?

The basic difference is in how quickly they take effect, so they can be divided into short-, medium- or long-acting varieties. The short-acting insulin is always clear or colourless, whereas the other two are cloudy because they contain additives to slow down the absorption of insulin from under the skin. It is possible to mix short- and medium-acting insulins in the same syringe, but care must be taken not to contaminate the clear insulin with any cloudy insulin. For this reason the clear is always drawn up first.

If you find it difficult to mix insulins yourself, you may be able to use one of the ready-mixed kinds which contain quick- and medium-acting insulins in different proportions.

All three types of insulin may be produced from animal sources – pig or beef – or from genetically engineered human hormone. Some so-called human insulin is in fact derived originally from pigs but altered so that it is indistinguishable from the human version. Human insulin is the most widely pre-scribed insulin in the UK.

Is human insulin better than pig or beef?

This is a controversial area and some patients who changed from animal to human insulin have said that they feel less well since the switch. It seems that human insulin is absorbed slightly more quickly from under the skin. However, no measurable differences in blood glucose levels have been found when human and animal insulins were tested under control conditions. Nevertheless, some people do prefer the animal preparations, and at the moment supplies are still available and said to be guaranteed for the foreseeable future.

Why do I have to inject insulin several times a day?

The object of insulin therapy is to imitate the body's natural supply as

BLOOD GLUCOSE AND INSULIN LEVELS IN NON-DIABETIC AND DIABETIC PEOPLE TAKING INSULIN

Normal condition

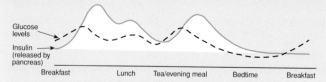

In a person who doesn't have diabetes, insulin is released by the pancreas in response to food.

Multiple injections (basal-bolus) reproduce normal condition

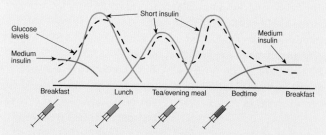

Many people inject themselves with short-acting insulin three times a day before meals in addition to a night-time injection of medium- or long-acting insulin to control blood glucose overnight. Meal times are flexible with this method.

Twice daily injections reproduce normal condition

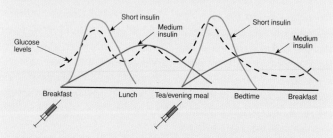

Two injections a day of short- and medium-acting insulins cover the meal you are about to have as well as a later meal or over night. Meal timing is important to avoid low glucose levels.

closely as possible. In a person who doesn't have diabetes, insulin is released by the pancreas in response to food (see diagram on page 24). As the blood glucose level falls between meals, so the insulin level drops back towards zero. It never quite gets there, however, and there is no time in the 24 hours when there is no detectable insulin in the bloodstream. What you are trying to do when you give yourself insulin injections is to reproduce the normal pattern of insulin production from the pancreas.

There are several ways of doing this using different types of insulin and numbers of injections per day. For example, many people follow a system which comprises three injections of short-acting insulin before the three main meals of the day, plus a night-time injection of a medium- or long-acting insulin to control blood glucose while they're asleep. Another popular and equally successful system involves two injections a day of a mixture of short- and medium-acting insulins. The idea is that the short-acting component covers the meal you're about to have (say breakfast or tea/evening meal), while the medium-acting component covers you at lunchtime or overnight. Many people have been using one or other of these systems very happily for years, and the choice between them is often simply a matter of personal preference.

If you're one of the relatively few people who simply can't get used to giving yourself several injections a day, or if you have only a partial failure of your insulin supply, you may be able to make do with just one or two daily injections of medium- or long-acting insulin.

How and where do I inject myself?

Your diabetes care team will show you how to do the injections and explain the various types of equipment available. Many people today use disposable plastic syringes and needles, although a few still prefer the old-style glass ones with disposable needles. Disposable syringes and needles can be used many times with little risk of infection. They are usually thrown away when the needle becomes blunt and injections become less comfortable.

Insulin injection pens are also very popular, largely because of their convenience and portability. Although the pens themselves are free, the needles still have to be paid for, although there is currently an active campaign to try to persuade the Department of Health to allow free prescription of pen needles. There are several types of pen to choose from, but the principles of the device are much

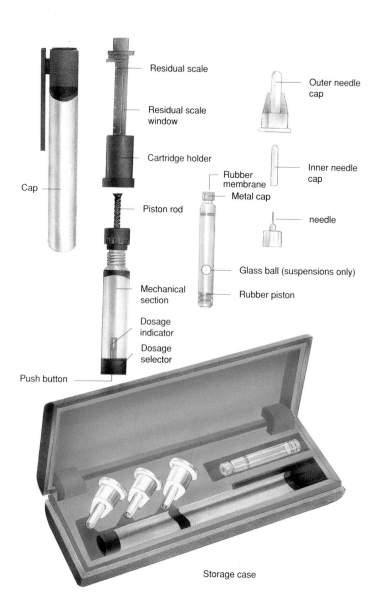

Residual scale

Residual scale window

Cartridge holder

Piston rod

Mechanical section

Dosage indicator

Dosage selector

Push button

Cap

Outer needle cap

Inner needle cap

needle

Rubber membrane

Metal cap

Glass ball (suspensions only)

Rubber piston

Storage case

A typical insulin injection pen.

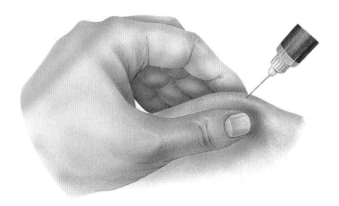

Pinch the skin and inject the bunched up area at an angle of 90°.

the same (see page 26). It's simply a matter of which one suits you best.

As we've already seen, you inject insulin under your skin rather than into a vein or muscle. Recent research has suggested that many people may have been getting the depth wrong so that insulin is going into the muscle beneath the skin by mistake.

Judging the depth accurately can be quite difficult, especially if you're slim, but it's important to master the technique because insulin can be absorbed from muscle more rapidly than expected. Your diabetes care team will show you how to do it properly, but a lot of people find that the simplest way is to pinch the skin and inject the bunched up area at an angle of 90 degrees. Don't pinch too hard though or it will hurt when the needle goes in! For patients who

may be having difficulty with inadvertent muscular injection, there are different lengths of needle available and this problem should be discussed with your diabetes care team.

You'll be given advice about the best sites for injection (see page 28). The tops of the thighs, buttocks and abdomen are the most common sites, and it's best to avoid using the same area every time, otherwise you could develop a small fatty lump (called lipo-hypertrophy) which could affect the smoothness of insulin absorption.

It's probably a good idea to inject medium- or longer-acting insulins into your thigh or buttock and use your tummy for quick-acting injections, but the most important thing is that you should be happy about the sites you're using.

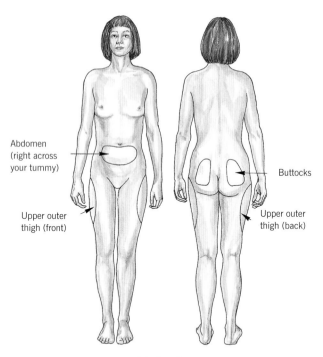

Abdomen
(right across
your tummy)

Buttocks

Upper outer
thigh (front)

Upper outer
thigh (back)

Injection sites.

Will the injections hurt or mark?

People who've been giving themselves injections for years say they don't feel a thing, but many beginners may find it slightly painful at first. Try to be as relaxed as you can and follow the technique you've been shown. Some people find it helps to rub the skin with ice for a few seconds beforehand to numb it, and you might like to give this a try.

As you get more practice, you should find that the injections rarely hurt, but if things don't improve, it's worth asking someone at the diabetes care centre for advice on what's causing the problem.

The needles are very fine and usually do not leave a mark. Sometimes you may get a little bleeding after an injection or even a bruise, but this is nothing to worry about. It just means you've probably punctured one of the tiny blood vessels under the skin, and this happens from time to time. There is virtually no chance of insulin directly entering the bloodstream, so don't worry if you notice some bleeding.

KEY POINTS

✓ Tablet treatment is useful for type 2 patients

✓ Tablets work in different ways and have different side effects. Be sure to check these with your diabetes care team when they are prescribed

✓ Insulin injections are necessary for all type 1 and many type 2 patients

✓ At least two and maybe four injections are needed a day

✓ Injections rarely cause discomfort or leave any mark

✓ Insulin preparations can be short, medium or long acting

✓ New pre-mixed short- and medium-acting preparations are now available

Checking your glucose levels

The point of all treatment for diabetes – whether it's diet, tablets or insulin – is to keep the levels of glucose in your bloodstream as close as possible to normal. The nearer you get to achieving this, the better you will feel, especially in the long term. There are two ways you can monitor glucose levels for yourself and your doctor will advise you about which one you should use and how often to do the checks. The two methods available are blood tests and urine tests, and neither is particularly difficult once you get the hang of it.

The development of simple finger-prick blood testing methods in the last few years has transformed life for patients taking insulin. Keeping a close check on your glucose levels is very useful when you're on insulin because it means you can make adjustments to your dose depending on the results. When your diabetes is controlled by tablets and/or diet, urine tests can give you nearly as much information as blood tests and may be more convenient.

In addition, there are blood tests that can be performed in hospital which measure an average blood glucose level over a period before the test, which may be from two to eight weeks. We will look at each of these three approaches in turn.

BLOOD TESTS

There are two systems available for self blood glucose monitoring (or SBGM as you may hear it called). Both give accurate results, and as well as helping you improve your blood glucose control, they can be useful if you suspect you may be about to have a hypoglycaemic reaction (see page 36). Taking an exact reading will either reassure you that all is well or confirm that you need to take action. Blood testing strips are available on prescription but the special meters for reading them have to be purchased separately.

Method 1

The glucose in the drop of your blood reacts with a pad or pads on the end of a plastic strip. These pads have been impregnated with chemicals and form colours when exposed to glucose. These colours are then either matched against a chart on the side of the blood testing stick container or inserted into the appropriate meter which gives a more precise reading.

There are several different strips available, each of which has a different reaction time, so it is vital to follow the manufacturer's instructions carefully, otherwise your reading could be too high or too low.

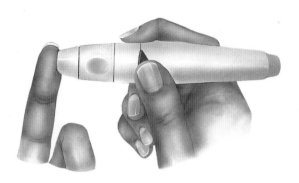

Spring-loaded lancet.

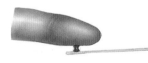

Match the colour on the strip with the colour chart on the container.

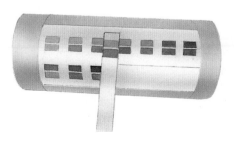

Checking blood glucose levels by matching colours.

Method 2: Medisense

A slightly more complicated chemical reaction takes place when the drop of your blood is put on the specially designed testing strip. There is no colour change involved and the strips can only be read using a special meter. This system needs slightly less blood than the conventional colour pad system, but the meters have to be purchased.

Pricking your finger

The main drawback for some people is that both these systems mean you have to obtain a finger-prick sample of your own blood (although occasionally someone else may be able to do this for you). Pricking your finger can be especially difficult if you are a manual worker or if you have very sensitive fingers. Rather than having to nerve yourself deliberately to stab your finger, you might find it easier to use one of the devices that incorporates a spring-loaded lancet. It allows you to adjust the depth of the prick to suit yourself, but the disadvantage is that, although the lancets are available on prescription, the spring-loaded devices have to be paid for.

URINE TESTS

Glucose appears in your urine when your kidneys can no longer reabsorb the amount being filtered. The problem with urine testing is that this 'overflow point' isn't the same for everyone. The correct term for this overflow point is the kidney (or renal) threshold. Some people who don't have diabetes have a low

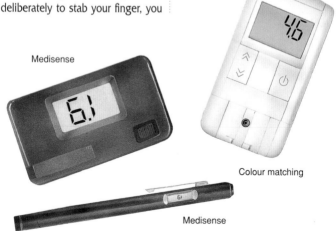

Medisense

Colour matching

Medisense

Examples of blood glucose meters.

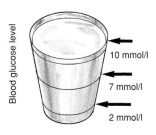

Kidney (or renal) threshold for glucose. Imagine this bucket is your kidneys. They can only cope with a maximum blood level of glucose and if the bucket overflows glucose appears in your urine.

threshold, and they often need the glucose tolerance test described on page 8 to confirm the fact and explain why glucose has appeared in their urine.

The normal threshold is around a blood glucose level of 10 millimoles per litre (mmol/l), so for a person with diabetes, a negative urine test can mean your blood glucose level is anywhere between 0 and 10 mmol/l, depending on your personal threshold. A positive test, on the other hand, doesn't tell you the exact level of blood glucose or by how much it exceeds your own personal threshold.

Despite this relative lack of accuracy, however, testing your urine and getting mostly negative results may be all you need to confirm that you have your diabetes well under control, especially if you're being treated with diet and/or tablets.

How to do it

Nearly everyone these days uses stick tests similar to those used for testing blood glucose. You dip a stick either into the stream of urine or into a specimen you've just passed, then wait for the chemical reaction which results in a colour change. You then read off the colour against the chart which is usually printed on the side of the container. As with the blood testing sticks, how long you wait varies from one type of urine stick to another, so do check the manufacturer's instructions.

The test must be done on fresh urine if it is to reflect the level of glucose in your blood at the time it's done. This is especially important first thing in the morning, when urine may have been accumulating in your bladder over several hours. What you have to do is empty your

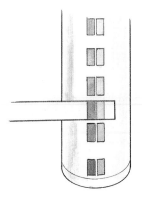

Urine test.

bladder about half an hour before you want to do the test, then pass another sample about half an hour later which is the one you actually check.

WHAT THE RESULTS TELL YOU

When you do either a blood or a urine test, you're really measuring how effective your previous dose of insulin or tablet treatment has been. In other words, doing a test just before lunch will tell someone on insulin the effect of their early morning injection of quick-acting insulin. In the same way, a pre-breakfast test will reflect the effectiveness of the previous night-time dose. The same interpretation applies in principle to tablets.

When the test result shows a high level of glucose, you may have to increase the size of your next dose of medication to restore the balance. This solves the problem short term, but ideally you want to prevent the problem arising in the first place by adjusting the dose which preceded the test. It's a good idea to vary the time of day when you do your test, and also to wait for a series of results over a period of, say, three to five days, before making too many adjustments. That way, you will see whether there is any pattern to the changes in your blood glucose level.

Until you have more experience of handling your diabetes, it would be better to consult your GP or someone in your diabetes care team before altering your insulin or tablet dosage. Later on, once you've learned more about your body's reactions, you'll be able to make the necessary adjustments on your own because you'll know what works for you.

HOSPITAL MONITORING

If you have type 1 diabetes, there may be situations where your medical advisers feel it would be useful to assess the effectiveness of your treatment by means of more sophisticated blood tests. They are not a substitute for your own routine testing, but can give additional information which will help the doctor decide whether your treatment needs adjustment. Both tests require a blood sample to be taken from a vein.

Glycated haemoglobin

This measures your average blood glucose level over a period of some six to eight weeks. Like all averages, however, it could be the result of lots of small variations or much larger swings in either direction. For this reason, it isn't useful for making day-to-day adjustments of insulin treatment, but is a good guide as to whether your treatment is working well overall.

Fructosamine

This test works on the same principle as glycated haemoglobin, but measures treatment effectiveness over a shorter period – around the previous two to three weeks. Again it is a useful guide as to whether your current treatment is working well or needs adjustment.

KEY POINTS

✓ Blood tests provide more accurate information about glucose control

✓ Blood tests are more helpful to exclude hypoglycaemia (low blood glucose)

✓ Urine tests are perfectly adequate for monitoring patients on diet control or low doses of OHAs, but are not very helpful for alerting the patient to hypoglycaemia

All about hypoglycaemia

You only need to be concerned about 'hypos' if you are being treated with insulin or sulphonylurea tablets. If your diabetes is controlled just by diet or you are taking metformin or acarbose, you will not experience this problem. Hypoglycaemia means low blood glucose, and in a person who doesn't have diabetes, the levels never fall much below 3.5 mmol/l. This is because their natural control system will sense the drop, and correct the situation by stopping insulin secretion and releasing other hormones such as glucagon which boost blood glucose. What's more, the person will start to feel hungry, and so do the right thing by eating, so raising their blood glucose.

When you're on insulin or sulphonylureas, this feedback system no longer operates. Once you have taken insulin or stimulated its production with tablets, you can't switch it off again, so your blood glucose will go on dropping until you have some food in the form of carbohydrate. As the level falls, it usually triggers a variety of warning symptoms (see box). Hypoglycaemia is dangerous because the brain is almost entirely dependent on glucose for normal functioning. If levels drop too low, the brain starts to work less well and produces the symptoms shown in the box. If the level drops even lower unconsciousness (coma) may result.

PREVENTING HYPOS

In past years, someone who was being started on insulin might have had to go through a deliberately induced hypoglycaemic reaction so he or she would know how it felt. These days your doctor is unlikely to suggest this as it's not very pleasant! Doing a blood glucose test at home means you can find out quickly and easily whether your level is getting too low and take action if necessary.

One of the most important aspects of caring for patients with diabetes is trying to ensure that they don't suffer from hypoglycaemic reactions. This involves the individual concerned discussing their treatment and adjusting it if necessary to fit in with their lifestyle, especially with their meal and work patterns. This is not always easy, and sometimes it means compromises will have to be worked out. You usually have to accept that there is no alternative to sticking to regular mealtimes, however inconvenient you find it. However, with the wide range of different insulins and types of injection device, it is usually possible to arrive at a treatment programme that will suit you.

HYPOGLYCAEMIA: YOUR SYMPTOM CHECKLIST

- Feeling sweaty or cold and clammy
- Trembling and feeling weak
- Tingling around your lips
- Feeling hungry
- Blurred vision
- Feeling irritable, upset or angry
- Unable to concentrate
- Looking pale
- Feeling drowsy (and losing consciousness if nothing is done)

Sometimes, people suffering from low blood glucose may behave oddly, so that others suspect them of being drunk. Most people who are taking insulin can use their symptoms as a signal that they need to have some food fairly quickly. However, just which symptoms you get and how severe they are is an individual thing – some people feel hungry before noticing anything else, others experience tingling round the lips or shakiness, for example. You may not experience all of these symptoms, however, but it is usual to have a headache after a 'hypo'.

Having regular hypoglycaemic attacks is a sign that you need to go back to your doctor or nurse to see how your treatment and/or your eating pattern can be adjusted to prevent them happening.

WHAT CAUSES HYPOS?

You'll soon get to recognise the situations where you are especially vulnerable, but the most common are:

- Eating later than you had expected or planned, which is bound to happen sometimes. If you've had your insulin injection and then can't eat for some reason, you should eat a small carbohydrate snack (such as a boiled sweet or a biscuit), which you ought to have handy at all times.

- A burst of unexpected exercise – such as running for a bus (for more on this, see page 42).

- Drinking too much alcohol. When your liver has to break down excessive quantities of alcohol, it can't produce glucose at the same time. This is why you'll be advised not to drink too much if you're on insulin or taking sulphonylureas and always to eat something whenever you do have an alcoholic drink.

TREATING A HYPO

A reaction that's relatively mild can usually be dealt with quite simply – a glass of Lucozade or lemonade should do the trick. Remember, though, that diet drinks contain artificial sweetener rather than sugar, so are of no use to you in this situation. Do make sure too that, wherever you are, you always carry some sort of readily available carbohydrate in the form of a boiled sweet or a biscuit. This is especially important if you're a driver or if you're about to take some form of vigorous exercise. For more on this, see the sections on diet (page 10) and exercise (page 42).

WHEN IT'S SEVERE

Very occasionally, you may find that your blood glucose level drops so rapidly that you don't have time to take the corrective action described above. You may become drowsy or unconscious, and might even have an epileptic fit. This is obviously a frightening prospect both for you and for those close to you, and you need to take action to make sure it doesn't happen again. This means getting advice from your medical team to get the problem sorted out. There are various ways of dealing with a person who's having a severe hypo.

- When you're not in a state to eat or drink anything, a sugary gel called Hypostop can be squirted into your mouth or rubbed on your gums. *This should not be done if the person is having a fit.*

- A hormone called glucagon which causes blood glucose to rise is available in injectable form. You can be given an injection into your arm or buttock to bring you round, so you can then have something to eat or drink.

NIGHT-TIME HYPOS

It's natural for you and your family to worry that you might have a hypo while you're asleep, or even that you might have one and not wake up. This is an especially frightening prospect when you are the parent of a small child with type 1 diabetes – for more on this, see page 50.

In reality, the problem is by no means as dramatic as that. First, you are quite likely to be woken up by the symptoms of falling blood glucose. You may feel sweaty, restless or irritable. Occasionally, your restlessness may wake your partner even if you stay asleep. It's not unusual to sleep right through a severe hypoglycaemic reaction. Your body mobilises various hormones in response to the falling level of glucose which will stimulate the release of stored glucose to correct the situation. After a

reaction like this, you'll wake up with a headache and symptoms much like a bad hangover. Sometimes, there may be a swing too far in the opposite direction, so that your blood glucose rises too far. If you regularly wake up feeling bad with these sort of symptoms it's a good idea to take a few early morning (2 to 4 a.m.) blood glucose tests to see if you are having hypoglycaemic reactions which you're not aware of at the time. At least then you'll know why you're feeling so bad and you need to talk to your doctor about whether your night-time dose of insulin needs adjusting or altering to a different type.

HYPOGLYCAEMIC AWARENESS

You may well have read various stories about some people with diabetes complaining that they have lost their 'early warning system' of a hypoglycaemic reaction. Many of them believe that this has happened as a result of changing from animal to human insulin. Before we consider this aspect, we should look at other reasons why this awareness might be lost.

It has become increasingly clear for some years that people who have had diabetes for a very long time become less able to predict when they are about to have a hypo. The warning signs seem to become less noticeable after they've been on insulin for about 15 to 20 years. Although no one knows quite why this should be so, it is true that the ability of the pancreas to release glucagon in response to low blood glucose diminishes over time. Some people say their symptoms change, while others say they come on so much faster that they don't have time to take corrective action. The problem is also more common in people whose average blood glucose levels are on the low side of normal. Sometimes, adjusting the treatment so as to allow the blood glucose level to rise slightly may mean the person gets their old pattern of symptoms back, but any change of this kind must be discussed carefully with the diabetes care team.

The question of what role human insulin may play in changing awareness is even more complex. While some patients feel that changing from animal insulin is responsible for their difficulties,

HAVING A HYPO

This is when the blood glucose level of a person on insulin or sulphonylurea tablets drops too low.

Possible causes:

- A delayed or missed meal or snack
- More exercise than usual – including things like gardening, strenuous housework or sport
- An illness that means you eat less than usual

Treatment:

1 Take some quick-acting carbohydrate, such as glucose tablets or a glucose drink
2 As soon after as you can, have some slower-acting carbohydrate such as sandwiches or toast
3 Check your blood glucose if possible
   Take more glucose if your symptoms persist
   If you're due to have a meal or a snack, eat something as soon as you can
   If your symptoms still don't go, seek medical advice

their doctors often disagree. Carefully controlled experiments have shown no measurable difference in hypoglycaemic symptoms in people taking animal or human insulin. All the same, some people are quite sure that they feel better on animal insulin, and if so, there is absolutely no reason why they shouldn't go on taking it.

Can hypoglycaemia be avoided by constant high blood glucose levels?

Having persistently high blood glucose levels will avoid hypoglycaemia, but unfortunately increases the risk dramatically of developing complications of diabetes (see page 54). Maintaining the balance between risky hyperglycaemia and troublesome hypoglycaemia can be very difficult for patients on insulin, but is much easier these days with the different preparations and injection devices available. If you are having troublesome hypo attacks, followed by high blood glucose levels, please consult your diabetes care team as it may mean that your treatment needs adjusting or changing.

KEY POINTS

✓ Hypoglycaemia can occur in any patient taking insulin or sulphonylurea tablets

✓ Individual patients differ in their warning signs of hypoglycaemia

✓ If you think a hypo may be coming on, try to confirm with a blood test first

✓ If this is not possible take some fast-acting carbohydrate such as Lucozade or lemonade (not low calorie)

✓ Milk and biscuits are not ideal because they are not rapidly absorbed

✓ If hypoglycaemia is a recurrent problem, seek advice from your diabetes care team

Breaking your routine

EXERCISE

When a person who doesn't have diabetes takes exercise, the release of insulin from the pancreas is shut down, while other hormones are produced which cause the blood glucose level to rise. When you're taking insulin or sulphonylurea tablets, however, your insulin level goes on rising, and if you've had an injection into one of the limbs you're exercising, the insulin may be absorbed faster than usual. It's important to let the people you're with – say, your tennis partner or the other members of a football team – know when you're taking insulin and explain to them what to do if you have a hypoglycaemic reaction.

When you know you're going to exercise, you can adjust your medication and/or your diet to make allowances. Your dose of insulin may have to be cut by as much as a half, depending on how vigorous an exercise session you're planning. It's more difficult when you take exercise unexpectedly, and this can be a particular problem

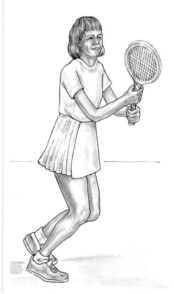

It's important to let the people you're with know when you're taking insulin and explain to them what to do if you have a hypo.

with children. Once again, the solution is to have your quick-acting carbohydrate snack handy – a drink, a biscuit or even a bar of chocolate.

As long as you take sensible precautions, there's no reason at all why you shouldn't take part in any kind of sport that you want to and at any level. Both Gary Mabbutt and Alan Kernaghan have type 1 diabetes and played Premier League football. Many people with diabetes take part in just about every known sport – although there are some which require special considerations, such as scuba diving or hang gliding and they might be better avoided! In any case, the high-risk sports often have special rules and regulations relating to people with diabetes, and it is important for your own safety that you abide by them.

PARTY TIME

With a little thought and pre-planning, you can feel free to go to any party and enjoy yourself as much as ever. The main considerations are that you will probably be eating later than usual, having different kinds of food and possibly dancing late into the night. When you're on insulin, you will need to make certain adjustments to take account of these factors. When you know you're going to be having a meal several hours later than normal, have a light snack before you go, then delay your injection until the food is ready.

If the party starts really late, you'll probably need extra carbohydrate with your meal along with your normal insulin dose. Take some extra food with you – and perhaps some Lucozade too – if you plan to keep going into the small hours. The best plan for those on a basal-bolus regimen is to substitute the overnight medium-acting insulin with a smaller dose of quick-acting insulin plus a snack at around

REMEMBER:

- When you're treated with tablets, you'll need to eat more to allow for extra activities such as dancing.
- Never drink alcohol on an empty stomach; always have some carbohydrate first.
- Keep some quick-acting carbohydrate with you on a crowded dance floor in case of hypoglycaemia. It may not be possible to get to a bar or eating area quickly enough.

midnight. A blood test around three or four hours later is a good idea if you can manage it. Dancing will mean you have to have extra carbohydrate – how much depends on how much energy you put into your performance!

WHEN YOU'RE TRAVELLING

There's no reason why your diabetes should interfere with or restrict your travel plans in any way, although if you're going abroad, you'd be wise to take out comprehensive travel insurance. Medical care and treatment abroad is rarely free, although the UK does have reciprocal arrangements with some other countries.

If you're going to one of the countries of the European Union, you should complete form E111 (from DSS offices or main post offices) and obtain a certificate before you go. Even when a country does offer a reciprocal scheme, it's still worth having your own insurance on top, and essential in those countries where the health care is not equivalent to that provided by the NHS or is very expensive (the USA, for instance).

There may be special considerations when you're heading somewhere extremely remote or inaccessible – so discuss your plans with your diabetes care team. Wherever you're going, and especially if it's off the beaten track, make sure that

you will be able to obtain insulin or tablets there if necessary, just in case you somehow get parted from your own supplies. Never pack all your insulin in your suitcase!

You'll need to check out the immunisation requirements for your destination well in advance – sometimes it takes several weeks to complete the course. Preventive measures of this kind may be particularly important for travellers with diabetes, and it is reassuring to know that taking antimalarial tablets will not interfere with treatment for diabetes.

CROSSING TIME ZONES

You need to plan carefully if you're going on a long flight, and it's a good idea to do this with the help of your doctor or diabetes care team. Remember that travelling west extends your day, while travelling east shortens it.

• **When you're on insulin**: You will have fewer problems if you're on a multiple basal-bolus regimen using an injection pen than if you normally inject just twice a day. For an extended day, the simplest solution is to have an extra injection of quick-acting insulin before the extra meal that's almost bound to be given during your flight. When you reach your destination, have your normal evening dose of insulin followed by your evening meal.

Next morning, have your insulin before breakfast as usual, then try to match your eating pattern to that of the locals, although this isn't always easy if you have jet lag!

The night will probably be shorter when you're travelling east, so you should have a smaller dose of medium-acting insulin (perhaps 10–20 per cent less than usual), either before your evening meal if you're on twice-daily injections or before bed if you're on multiple injections, followed by your usual pre-breakfast dose next day.

Don't forget that you're not obliged to eat all the meals offered on the flight if you feel you don't want or need them. It is important to let the airline staff know that you have diabetes, and make sure they or your travelling companions know what to do if you have a hypo-glycaemic reaction and how to give insulin if you need it. The same applies if you're travelling by sea.

You don't have to have a fridge to store your insulin as long as you can keep it somewhere relatively cool, but if this is likely to be a problem, use a wide-necked vacuum flask.

• **When you're on tablets**: You shouldn't need to make any particular changes to your treatment schedule, but it would still be worth getting the advice of your doctor before taking a very long flight.

BE PREPARED

You will have to find room in your hand luggage for your medication, blood glucose testing equipment and any other medical kit; luggage does sometimes go missing! When you're carrying syringes and needles, it's sometimes useful to have a letter from your doctor on headed paper explaining that you have diabetes and how it is treated. This is important if you're going to some Middle and Far Eastern countries. It's also advisable for anyone with diabetes to carry some form of ID card or bracelet indicating that you have the condition and what medication you take. The British Diabetic Association (see page 74) can supply ID cards giving details of your treatment in the local language of the country you're going to and it's worth getting one of these. You may never need to show anyone either of these, but it won't hurt to have them, just in case.

Dose Card

I AM A DIABETIC
Name _____
Address _____
Telephone _____
Dose _____

It's quite safe to take travel sickness remedies along with your diabetes treatment if you need to,

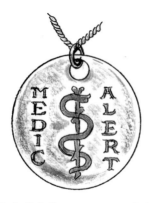

Medic-Alert offer an emergency medical information service 24 hours a day. See page 74.

but if you know you're prone to suffer in this way, take a supply of fruit juice or other sweet drink in case you can't eat much.

In other respects, you only need to follow the same commonsense rules as any other traveller – make sure you don't have too much sun, check out the alcohol content of unfamiliar local drinks and try to steer clear of unhygienic cafes or food-stalls!

WHEN YOU'RE NOT WELL

Everyone gets colds and 'flu from time to time, and these, like other illnesses, can affect the control of your diabetes. The most likely result is that your blood glucose level will rise, so you need to make frequent checks to test whether this is happening, especially if you are on insulin.

Type 1 (IDDM)

Many people think that if they're not eating they shouldn't take their insulin, otherwise they will have a hypo. In fact, the opposite is the case. Your blood glucose level is much more likely to be too high than too low in these circumstances. Even if you have a stomach bug such as gastroenteritis and are being sick all the time, you will still need some insulin to keep your glucose under control. If you can't keep any fluids down, you must call your doctor straightaway. You may have to go into hospital for a while until you are able to eat and drink again.

Type 2 (NIDDM)

Continuing to take your tablets when you're not able to eat or drink may cause a hypoglycaemic reaction. You may need a lower dose while you're ill, but unless you're monitoring your blood glucose regularly, you may need your doctor's advice on how to make the adjustment. If your illness doesn't settle down quickly, you may be admitted to hospital for a few days.

HAVING A BABY

The fact that you have diabetes is no reason to put off having a baby. The condition does not affect your fertility, and you should have no problems conceiving unless you are one of the minority of women who have severe complications or whose diabetes is poorly controlled.

If you are planning to conceive in the near future, it's a good idea to make sure that your blood glucose levels are as well controlled as possible. In addition, folic acid supplements are highly recommended. You should ideally talk this over with your diabetes care team – you may find that your hospital offers a special preconceptual counselling service.

You need to watch your blood glucose levels particularly carefully when you're pregnant because, if they get too high, they can affect the baby. This can mean the baby grows too quickly or that too much fluid accumulates in the surrounding membranes. Your doctor will probably want to see you every few weeks, and you'll also be asked to do your own blood glucose checks more often than usual. It's likely that your insulin dose will double or even treble during this time, but

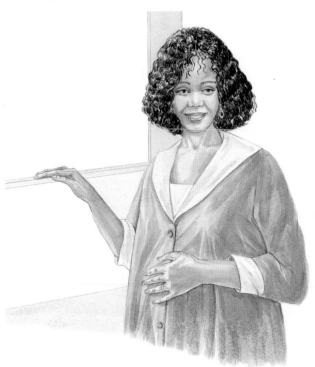

You can enjoy a healthy pregnancy and a normal healthy baby at the end of it.

they'll go back to normal after the birth. The insulin can't do your baby any harm, as it does not seem to lower the baby's blood glucose, and there's no need to worry either that you could injure him or her by injecting into your abdomen. Hypoglycaemia is not known to harm the baby in any way.

There's a good chance that you will be able to have a normal delivery, although some women do have to have a caesarean section. This is because some babies from diabetic mothers whose glucose levels were higher than ideal may have grown too large for normal vaginal delivery. Your obstetric and diabetes care teams will discuss the options with you beforehand, and if a normal delivery is decided on, you may well have a drip containing insulin and a sugar solution to control your diabetes during labour.

Huge advances in the antenatal care of women with diabetes in recent years mean that you can look forward to a healthy pregnancy and a normal, healthy baby at the end of it.

Gestational diabetes

Some women develop diabetes for the first time when they're pregnant, after which their blood glucose levels return to normal. Usually, gestational diabetes, as it's known, can be kept under control by eating the right kinds of foods, although some women do have to have insulin injections. You won't be treated with tablets while you're pregnant. After the birth, you'll be advised to keep an eye on your weight and stick to a healthy diet because you are at a greater than normal risk of developing type 2 diabetes later in life.

It's important to let the people you're with know when you're taking insulin and explain to them what to do if you have a hypo.

KEY POINTS

✓ If planning vigorous excercise, remember to take extra carbohydrate or reduce your insulin or sulphonylurea medication beforehand

✓ If exercising with others, always tell them that you have diabetes and explain what to do in the event of a hypoglycaemic attack

✓ For parties remember never to drink alcohol on an empty stomach and have some quick-acting carbohydrate always available

✓ If eating later than usual or having extra food you may need more insulin

✓ Remember to take out health insurance before any foreign travel

✓ If travelling between continents, heading west have an extra dose of insulin with your extra meal and heading east you may omit a scheduled meal and insulin dose

✓ Never pack your insulin in your suitcase

✓ Always carry identification stating your diagnosis and medication

✓ Even if you are ill and not eating, you still need your insulin or tablet medication

✓ If you cannot take your medication or insulin because of vomiting, seek medical help

✓ Diabetic women should try, wherever possible, to plan their pregnancy and seek early obstetric and medical advice once they realise that they are pregnant

Children with diabetes

Insulin-dependent (type 1) diabetes most commonly comes on between the ages of 11 and 13. It's quite unusual in children under five, although there have been cases of babies developing it within a few days of birth. You can't stop children racing around and burning up energy, which can make it difficult to keep their eating and insulin in the right balance. The usual answer is to give two or three injections a day each containing some short-acting and some medium-acting insulin. It's only to be expected that you'll worry about your child having hypoglycaemic reactions and find it hard to let him or her out of your sight. As they get older and you both get more used to dealing with diabetes you'll probably find it easier to allow them more independence.

Children can learn to inject themselves from any age, although you will probably want to check the insulin doses. Injector pens have been a big help in getting round this problem, because of their convenience and ease of dialling the insulin dose.

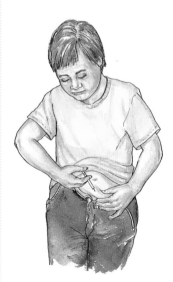

Children can learn to inject themselves but you will probably want to check the insulin doses.

HOME MONITORING

Blood tests can be hard for young children, and quite difficult because their fingers are so small, so urine tests are often recommended instead, either on their own or combined with occasional blood tests. Once your child is a bit older, you will have to encourage him or her to be disciplined about monitoring their blood glucose levels on a regular basis.

However, don't be surprised if he or she is awkward about it. Rebellion is a natural part of growing up, and many teenagers go through a period of refusing to cooperate over this aspect of their diabetes care. This is a difficult situation to deal with, but it's best to steer clear of direct confrontation as much as you can. Remember that it's much more important for your child to keep taking insulin regularly than to perform lots of blood glucose tests.

HYPOGLYCAEMIA

Children's blood glucose can fall quite quickly, especially if they are active, so it may be difficult to spot the warning signs in time. Very young children may not recognise them at all. When the blood glucose drops so low that the child becomes drowsy or even unconscious, the best treatment is glucagon. It's always worth keeping a supply handy if you are looking after a young child with diabetes.

Once this treatment has worked, then the child needs to have some carbohydrate in the form of food or a sweet drink. As the problem is most likely to arise when the child is exercising, it's essential that a playgroup leader, teacher or whoever is in charge (or a friend if the children are unsupervised) knows exactly what to do if he or she does have a hypoglycaemic reaction. In any case, once your child starts school, it's important that the staff are aware that he or she has diabetes and know what to do should he or she have a hypoglycaemic reaction. You will also need to make sure that the kitchen staff are aware of the situation if your child has lunch there, so that he or she makes the appropriate food choices!

PROBLEMS WITH FOOD

The amount that a child eats can vary by as much as 50 per cent from one day to the next. If you've ever looked after young children, you'll know how difficult it is to persuade them to eat anything some days, and at other times you can't stop them eating constantly. This obviously makes life rather difficult for you if you have a child with diabetes. As a rule, your main priority is to give your child something to eat whenever he or she is hungry, even if this means having more than their diet says they should. As children get older, they need bigger doses of insulin, and positive urine tests or high blood glucose values mean they need more insulin rather than less food. Low blood glucose, on the other hand, can mean a child needs either less insulin or more food, and this will need to be discussed with his or her diabetes care team.

Many children break the rules and eat sweets or chocolate on the quiet. You shouldn't cut down on their normal food intake to try and compensate for these extra illicit carbohydrates, however. If your child is old enough to understand, try to explain calmly why cheating in this way will result in high blood glucose, and this, in turn, may lead to complications (see page 54). Talking the situation over together in a calm and measured way with plenty of time is probably the best approach.

Children with diabetes will need to take the same kind of precautions as adults when their normal routine is disrupted, say by travel or by illness (see pages 44 and 46). They will also have to learn how to take care of themselves when exercising, and follow the commonsense rules outlined on page 42. If you are in any doubt about how to handle any of these situations, the team at your child's diabetes clinic will be happy to advise you.

FAMILY REACTIONS

When a child with diabetes has brothers or sisters, they may become jealous of the amount of extra attention he or she gets because of their condition. Equally, the child himself or herself may resent the fact that he or she has to cope with diabetes when the others don't have to bother. It's important that all these feelings are brought out into the open and discussed by the whole family. Talking things over – at regular intervals if necessary – can help to clear the air, and may encourage your other children to become involved in watching for signs of hypo-glycaemia. If they're old enough and willing, you should teach them how to treat a hypoglycaemic reaction (see page 38).

One area of possible family contention is mealtimes – with complaints from those who don't have diabetes about having to eat healthy foods! The fact is, of course, that the kind of diet recommended for people with diabetes is the same one we should all be following. It's not much fun for the child who has diabetes if the others constantly eat forbidden treats like sweets and chocolate in front of him or her, so do what you can to discourage this. Again, talking the situation over and explaining the problem is the approach that's most likely to work, and if you can persuade other children to restrict their sweets intake, it will be good for their health too.

PLAYING UP

Many children quickly discover that being awkward about food is a great way to wind their parents up, and those who have diabetes are no exception. They may well realise that refusing to eat at mealtimes or having a hypoglycaemic reaction is a surefire way to get masses of attention. They may also refuse to do urine or blood glucose tests or even make up the results.

This is obviously worrying and frustrating for you as parents, and can cause great disruption to family life. It's not at all unusual, however, and you shouldn't feel guilty because you feel that you can't cope. Your diabetes care team will have seen this kind of problem many times before, and be able to offer help and advice. Sometimes it can be a good idea to bring in an outsider – a family friend or even a specially trained counsellor – who can help the child concerned to understand the effect their behaviour is having. It's important to understand that this may some-times be a child's way of expressing his or her own deep-seated worries about the diabetes.

KEY POINTS

✓ Diabetes most commonly comes on between the ages of 11 and 13

✓ Very young children may need to rely on urine tests but older children should be encouraged to use blood tests if possible

✓ Food battles are even more common and problematic with diabetic children because of the risk of hypoglycaemia

✓ Try to avoid confrontation, however, and if battles are causing family upset please discuss the issues with your diabetes care team

If it gets complicated

The first thing you need to know is that you will not inevitably develop complications simply because you have diabetes. Careful research has shown that the better your blood glucose control, the less likely you are to experience any. A large study in the USA (called the Diabetes Control and Complications Trial) has suggested that any improvement in blood glucose control will reduce your risk of developing complications. Knowing this helps many

AFFECTED ORGANS

When complications do arise, the organs most likely to be affected are:

- Eyes
- Kidneys
- Peripheral nerves in the arms, hands, legs and feet
- Skin
- Large blood vessels

The good news is that many of the possible problems can be treated, and often the treatment is most effective when the complications are picked up early on. This is why you will be asked to go for regular medical check-ups.

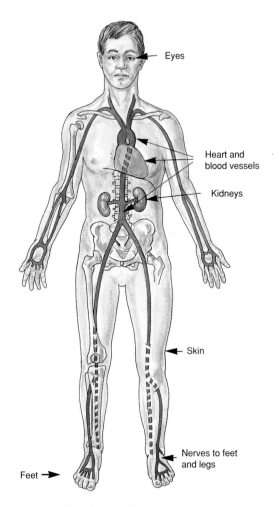

Eyes

Heart and
blood vessels

Kidneys

Skin

Nerves to feet
and legs

Feet

Sites of complications of diabetes.

people to work harder at controlling their diabetes when they're tempted to let things slide a little.

Along with good diabetic control, giving up (or not starting) smoking can reduce your chances of developing complications. Smoking and diabetes definitely don't mix. All of the possible complications listed below are more common in people who smoke, and anyone who has already developed any of them should stop smoking immediately. The importance of this can't be overstressed, and knowing that may be the incentive you need to help you give up if you are a smoker.

YOUR EYES

Diabetes can affect your eyes in various different ways.

Blurring

When you first start having insulin or tablet treatment, you may notice that your vision seems a bit blurred. This is because the lenses in your eyes became dehydrated when diabetes was developing, and by rapidly lowering your blood glucose, the treatment brings about a fluid shift into your eye. This is what causes any blurring. Fortunately, the problem is only temporary and should clear up in a few months without the need for treatment. If it happens to you, wait until the blurring has disappeared before getting a prescription for new glasses if you need one. The result of your sight test may well be different once your diabetes is stabilised.

Cataracts

When you have had diabetes for a long time, you are more susceptible to cataracts because of a build-up of sugars in the lens of the eye. These make the lens of your eye opaque, interfering with the transmission of light to the back of your eye, and can be a particular nuisance in bright sunlight. Fortunately, this problem can be treated quite easily with a simple operation to replace your damaged lens with a plastic

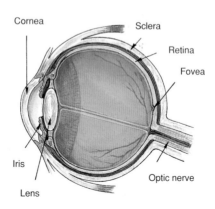

Cornea

Sclera

Retina

Fovea

Iris

Lens

Optic nerve

In the eye, it is the blood vessels supplying the retina which are mainly affected by diabetes.

one. It can often be done under a local anaesthetic, and you will normally only have to be in hospital for 24 hours. The results are generally excellent.

Retinopathy

Both types of diabetes can affect a highly specialised structure at the back of your eye called the retina. The central part (the macula) enables you to see colours and fine detail, while the outer (or peripheral) part picks up black and white and enables you to see in the dark.

It's the small blood vessels supplying the retina that are affected by diabetes. This is probably because of a build-up of glucose and other sugars in the walls of the blood vessels, making them weaker. Small blisters or microaneurysms can form and occasionally burst, resulting in tiny haemorrhages. Sometimes, blood vessels may leak, allowing fluid to collect on the surface of the retina, which then forms what are called hard exudates. This leakiness is usually a sign that the blood supply to that part of the eye is not as good as it should be. When retinopathy reaches an advanced stage, new blood vessels can grow as the body tries to improve the blood supply. These new vessels are fragile and may break and bleed extensively. This condition, known

as a vitreous haemorrhage, can seriously affect the sight.

Treating retinopathy

Fortunately, laser treatment developed in recent years can do a great deal to repair the damage caused by diabetic retinopathy. It's normally directed at the peripheral part of the retina, well away from the macula, and can remove hard exudates and prevent new blood vessels from growing. The earlier the treatment is given, the more successful it is, which is why it is essential that you should have your eyes checked at least once a year. Eye checks can be done by an optician, a specialist ophthal-mologist or a doctor who is skilled at this type of examination.

A few people may develop a more serious form of retinopathy called maculopathy, especially later in life. This means that the blood supply to the central part of the eye is reduced, which can seriously affect the person's ability to perceive colour and fine detail. Unfortunately, laser treatment is not so successful in treating this particular problem.

If you need laser treatment, you will normally be asked to attend the outpatient clinic at a special eye unit. First, drops are put into your eye to dilate the pupil so it's easier to see the retina. You then rest your head in a special bracket to keep it still while the doctor uses a type of camera to examine your eye and identify which parts of the retina need treatment. The treatment itself is usually painless, but you'll see brief flashes of bright light as the laser is used – sometimes several hundred in each treatment session. You may need several of these sessions for each eye, and afterwards, your vision could be blurred for about 24–48 hours.

YOUR KIDNEYS

The kidneys work as large blood filters, and one of their tasks is to get rid of excess water and the byproducts of everyday living. Diabetes can damage these filters, again by an accumulation of glucose in the tiny blood vessels that form them. The effect is similar to that of making the holes in a tea strainer larger. This damage allows substances which would normally be retained to pass into your urine.

One of the substances that appears in the urine when the filters are damaged is protein and a particular protein called albumin appears in the urine at a very early stage of diabetic kidney damage. Albumin in the urine is also called albuminuria and a current test can detect the presence of very small amounts (microalbuminuria). The availability of these tests is one reason why you will be asked to provide a urine sample at each of your diabetic clinic visits, even if you are normally performing blood tests for glucose. Sometimes you may get a positive result from the albumin test, which is in fact caused by a urinary infection. Your clinic will check your urine sample to exclude this.

Your doctor will want to keep a closer eye on you if albumin is detected in your urine because there is the possibility of more serious kidney damage and even kidney failure in the long term.

This is even more important if, like many people with albuminuria, you also have raised blood pressure. The two tend to go together because the kidneys also have a role in controlling blood pressure. Recent research has shown that treating high blood pressure in people with diabetes can dramatically slow down the effect of diabetes on their kidneys.

At the moment, those people who do eventually suffer from kidney failure may need treatment either by dialysis (a kidney machine) or by a transplantation, but there is a lot of research being done which may one day make this unnecessary.

YOUR NERVES

Diabetes can affect the nerves in two ways: as with the eyes and kidneys, their blood supply may be affected, or there can be direct damage to the nerves themselves as a result of high blood glucose.

Any kind of nerve damage is known medically as neuropathy. The consequences will depend on which of the three types of nerve is affected.

• **Motor nerves**: These carry messages to the muscles from the brain, stimulating them to contract. Damage to this type of nerve is known as motor neuropathy and can lead to a loss of small muscle activity in the feet or hands. As a result, the toes can become clawed and stick upwards, and the fingers become weak. For more on diabetes and the foot, see page 60.

• **Sensory nerves**: These detect pain, touch, heat and other sensations and send messages back to the brain. Sensory neuropathy can make the feet very sensitive and even painful at first, but eventually they will become numb and unable to feel any kind of sensation, including pain.

• **Autonomic nerves**: These are responsible for controlling automatic bodily functions such as bowel and bladder activity. Autonomic neuropathy is relatively uncommon, and its most troublesome effects are on the bladder and bowels. It can result in constipation or diarrhoea which comes and goes,

and occasionally the person may suffer from persistent vomiting. Men may also be troubled by a lowering of their sexual potency. Most of these problems can be improved by drug treatment.

SEXUAL POTENCY

A man's ability to have a normal erection depends upon a good supply of blood via the arteries to the penis, and on an intact nerve supply to constrict the veins leading from it. Blood enters the penis through the arteries, but cannot leave because the veins are constricted, thus producing an erection. Diabetes can affect both the blood supply and the nervous control needed to maintain an erection.

It's important to remember, however, that impotence can have psychological as well as physical causes, whether you have diabetes or not, so it's very important to discuss any sexual problems openly and frankly with your medical advisers. There are treatments available for all forms of sexual impotence in men.

YOUR SKIN

A small minority of people with diabetes may have skin problems caused by damage to the small blood vessels. When this occurs, it results in reddening and thinning of the skin over the lower shin bones –

a condition known as necrobiosis lipoidica. Unfortunately, there is no effective treatment.

YOUR ARTERIES

Your diabetes means you could be at increased risk of developing hardening of the large blood vessels or arteries, which can give rise to heart attacks and strokes, and also to poor circulation in the legs. Both smoking and being overweight increase the risk still more, so it is really essential that you avoid these. In any case, smoking is a known major risk factor for arterial disease even in people who don't have diabetes.

The problems caused by hardening of the arteries are very common, and there are both medical and surgical treatments available. However, it is well worth doing everything you can to prevent such problems developing in the first place.

YOUR FEET

You need to be aware of changes to your feet that can arise because of your diabetes and of what you can do to minimise the risk of damage. Most people with diabetes don't get serious foot problems, but even those who do can prevent things getting worse by caring for their feet properly. Healthy circulation to your feet will help to keep the tissues strong, and you can encourage this by eating the right kinds of foods, keeping good control of your diabetes and by not smoking. Ensure that your shoes fit well with enough room for your toes, and with a fastening to keep them in place without rubbing. In addition, there are specific things you can do to look after your feet.

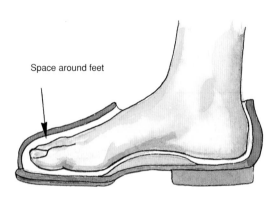

Space around feet

Avoid foot restriction.

These are designed to guard against four changes which can be caused by diabetes.

• **Poor blood supply**: The result of the blood vessels becoming narrower. When your circulation is restricted in this way, your foot is less able to cope with hazards like cold weather, infection or injury, and is more susceptible to the other three changes below. Keep your feet warm with good quality socks and stockings, but avoid over-heating and be very careful of seams in your socks that can press and rub, causing blisters. Consider wearing the socks inside out if the seams are prominent.

• **Neuropathy**: Neuropathy makes the foot less sensitive to pain and temperature. In its early stages, people often complain of pins and needles or a feeling that they are 'walking on cotton wool or pebbles'. When the ability of your foot to feel is reduced, you're less likely to notice accidental injuries or infection which will lead to increased damage if nothing is done. In some cases, skin breaks down over a part of the foot which has experienced sustained pressure, because you don't feel the discomfort that would otherwise make you shift your position.

If you are suffering from some degree of neuropathy, you have to get into the habit of checking your feet every day for any cuts or wounds which didn't hurt at the

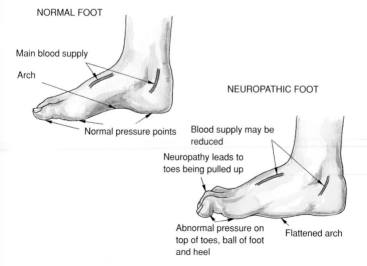

NORMAL FOOT

Main blood supply

Arch

Normal pressure points

NEUROPATHIC FOOT

Blood supply may be reduced

Neuropathy leads to toes being pulled up

Abnormal pressure on top of toes, ball of foot and heel

Flattened arch

time. The easiest way is to make a regular foot care programme part of your daily routine. It is also important to check the water temperature with your hand before getting into a bath, and to avoid 'toasting your toes' in front of the fire.

• **Dryness**: Loss of elasticity or dryness in the skin of your feet can be associated with neuropathy and a poor blood supply, but it can develop even when you have good circulation and a normal amount of feeling.

You may notice your skin is becoming dry even if you haven't had diabetes for very long, and be inclined to dismiss it as just a minor nuisance. However, dry and flaky skin is much less supple because it is not protected by sweat and

REMEMBER:

- Wash your feet daily in warm water using a mild soap. Don't soak them for a long time as it removes more of the precious oils from your skin. You may develop soggy areas between your toes which can split or increase the likelihood of soft corns.

- Apply surgical spirit to any white, damp areas between your toes, unless there has been any bleeding. If there has, use dry dressings instead. Any signs of athlete's foot can be treated with surgical spirit, but if that doesn't work, use an antifungal powder or spray from the chemist.

- Your toe nails should be cut or filed straight across, unless a state-registered chiropodist advises otherwise. Sharp corners can be filed over with a foot file or an emery board.

- Corns and calluses (hard skin) are best left to the state-registered chiropodist who will either provide or recommend specific protection for the affected areas. Lint pads or cushion soles may be useful temporary protection for affected areas if you can't get to see the chiropodist straight away.

- Get medical advice immediately if you see any signs of ulceration developing anywhere on your feet.

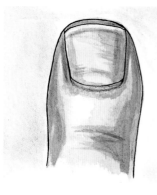

Nail cut correctly with cut made straight across, not protruding and not trimmed down the sides of the toe.

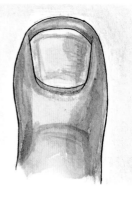

Nail cut incorrectly: too short and cut down each side

natural oils from the everyday pressures and frictions of walking. When the skin on your feet is very dry, you're more prone to the formation of calluses and corns, and also to splits around the edges (known as fissures).

You can help to replace some of the lost natural moisture by applying a good hand cream every day and using a foot file or pumice stone to remove dead skin. Do be gentle, though, and never, ever use chemicals designed to remove corns and calluses or try to cut them away with blades because you could easily injure yourself.

• **Changes in the shape of your feet**: These can take place over a period of time as a result of diabetes. The bones underneath may become more prominent due to changes in the fatty pad under the

ball of your foot. The front part of your foot may spread and your toes may claw. When the tissues under your foot are strained, you may get pain in your heel.

Usually, these changes are a result of minor alterations in the shape of your foot, but don't forget they could still mean you need new shoes to get a better fit.

EXPERT CARE

As a person with diabetes, you are eligible for treatment from a state-registered chiropodist (also called a podiatrist) on the NHS – your GP or health centre should have a list of local practitioners. Many people are perfectly able to look after their own feet, but anyone who has a physical or visual disability or any of the complications listed above should have regular appointments with a state-registered chiropodist.

Footnote!

You are probably feeling rather alarmed after reading about all these possible complications, so it's worth emphasising again that they can all be prevented by careful attention to diabetes care and blood glucose control.

Remember that complications are not inevitable – and that you have an important role in prevention.

KEY POINTS

✓ Diabetes can affect the eyes by causing cataracts or damage the back of the eyes – called retinopathy

✓ Early detection and treatment are very effective at preventing progression and loss of eye sight

✓ Kidney damage occurs in a minority of patients and can be detected early by a urine test for albumin

✓ Nerves can also be damaged and feet and hands need to be checked regularly

✓ Foot care is extremely important in preventing complications

✓ Feet should be inspected and washed daily and nails should be cut straight across with sharp edges smoothed off with a file

✓ Moisturisers can help prevent skin dryness

✓ Feet should be checked once a year by a health care professional

Who cares?

Medical and lay members of the British Diabetic Association (BDA) have drawn up a charter (see below) of what you should expect from your medical carers.

DIABETES CARE

What you should expect
When you have just been diagnosed, you should have:

- A full medical examination.

- A talk with a registered nurse who has a special interest in diabetes. She will explain what diabetes is and talk to you about your individual treatment.

- A talk with a state-registered dietitian, who will want to know what you are used to eating and will give you basic advice on what to eat in the future. A follow-up meeting should be arranged for more detailed advice.

- A discussion of the implications of your diabetes for your job, driving, insurance, prescription charges, etc. and whether you need to inform the DVLA and your insurance company, if you are a driver.

- Information about the BDA's services and details of your local BDA group.

- Ongoing education about your diabetes and the beneficial effects of exercise, and assessments of your control.

You should be able to take a close friend or relative with you to educational sessions if you wish.

If you are treated with insulin, you should have:

- Frequent sessions for basic instruction on injection technique, looking after insulin and syringes and pens, blood glucose testing and what the results mean.

- Supplies of relevant equipment.

- Discussion about hypoglycaemia (a hypo) and how to deal with it.

If you are treated by tablets, you should have:

- A discussion about the possibility of hypoglycaemia (a hypo) and how to deal with it.

- Instruction on blood or urine testing and what the results mean and supplies of relevant equipment.

If you are treated by diet alone, you should have:

- Instruction on blood or urine testing and what the results mean and supplies of relevant equipment.

Once your diabetes is reasonably controlled, you should:

- Have access to the diabetes

team at regular intervals – annually if necessary. These meetings should give time for discussion as well as assessing diabetes control.

- Be able to contact any member of the health care team for specialist advice when you need it.

- Have more education sessions as you are ready for them.

- Have a formal medical review once a year by a doctor experienced in diabetes.

At this review:

- Your weight should be recorded.

- Your urine should be tested for protein.

- Your blood should be tested to measure long-term control.

- You should discuss control, including your home monitoring results.

- Your blood pressure should be checked.

- Your vision should be checked and the back of your eyes examined. A photo may be taken of the back of your eyes. If necessary, you should be referred to an ophthalmologist.

- Your legs and feet should be examined to check your circulation and nerve supply. If necessary, you should be referred to a state-registered chiropodist.

- If you are on insulin, your injection sites should be examined.

- You should have the opportunity to discuss how you are coping at home and at work.

Your role
You are an important member of the care team, so it is essential that you understand your own diabetes to enable you to be in control of your own condition.

You should ensure you receive the described care from your local diabetes clinic, practice or hospital. If these services are not available, you should:

- Contact your GP to discuss the diabetes care available in your area

- Contact your local Community Health Council

- Contact the BDA or your local branch.

Questions & answers

Some questions come up time and again when people find out they have diabetes – here are the answers to some of the most common ones.

- Will I lose my driving licence because I have diabetes?

The short answer to this question is no. However, you do have to let the DVLA at Swansea know when your diabetes is first diagnosed, unless your treatment consists of diet alone. You'll find the address on your licence. The DVLA will issue you with a three-year licence; then, on the anniversary of renewal, you'll get a questionnaire from them to fill in. Depending on circumstances, you may be asked to see your GP or local diabetes clinic for a brief medical examination before your licence is renewed.

From January 1998, a European Community Directive on driving regulations came into effect. Motor vehicles are divided into four groups: groups A and B include motorcycles and motor vehicles under 3.5 tonnes in weight. These groups are not affected by the new regulations for diabetic patients.

However, groups C (motor vehicles over 3.5 tonnes but under 7.5 tonnes) and D (motor vehicles used for carrying passengers with more than eight but less than sixteen seats) will require a medical questionnaire to be completed. This has the same standards as the current LGV (large goods vehicle) and PCV (passenger-carrying vehicle) licences and all patients on insulin will be excluded from driving vehicles in these classes. There are apparently no exceptions to this, although the BDA and other groups are actively lobbying both the UK and European Parliaments to try to change the rules.

As well as the DVLA, you need

to let your motor insurance company know if your diabetes develops while the policy is in force. Some companies tend to load premiums for drivers with diabetes, and if this happens to you, contact the BDA (address on page 74) for their list of insurers offering preferential rates for drivers with the condition.

● Can I still enjoy a normal sex life?

Unless a man with diabetes has impotence problems, there is no reason why your sex life should be affected in any way and having diabetes makes no difference to a woman's fertility (see page 46). It's worth pointing out, though, that sexual intercourse is a vigorous activity and so could cause your blood glucose level to drop and precipitate a hypoglycaemic reaction.

● Can diabetes affect my job?

It depends to some extent on what you do. The main factor to consider, if you are on insulin or sulphonylureas, is what the consequences would be for both yourself and your colleagues if you suffered a hypoglycaemic reaction. For this reason, you would have to think carefully about whether to take up a job that involves physical hazards – such as working at heights like a steeplejack

or scaffolder – or other dangers, in the police or ambulance services, for example. However, if you're already employed in one of these areas when your condition is first diagnosed, you may be able to carry on if your diabetes is well controlled and you rarely experience hypoglycaemic reactions.

Whatever you do, it is important to tell your employer and your colleagues that you have diabetes, however tempting it might be to keep quiet. It could be very embarrassing and possibly dangerous for you and everyone else if you were to have a hypoglycaemic reaction and no one recognised it or knew what to do.

● Will my children get diabetes?

For insulin-dependent diabetic patients (type 1), there is a small but increased risk of their children also being affected. For unknown reasons, this is more likely if the father has diabetes, as opposed to the mother. If both parents have diabetes the risk is increased further. At present estimates the risk for a child with one parent with diabetes is around five per cent and if both parents have the condition it may be as high as 15 per cent.

For type 2 (NIDDM), the situation is much less clear. Some families with special types of diabetes have a very high risk of inheritance. These are, however, a very small minority and for most patients with type 2 diabetes the risk cannot be determined with any accuracy.

- Will I go blind or have kidney failure with diabetes?

As there is a tendency for diabetes to run in families, many patients have direct experience of relatives or acquaintances who have had severe complications from diabetes.

As far as eye and kidney problems are concerned these affect only a minority of patients and the risks of developing problems can be greatly reduced with careful control of blood glucose.

There are also many new treatments available for both eye and kidney complications which can prevent progression or deterioration provided the problem is picked up at an early stage. This is why it is critical that diabetic patients receive regular check-ups.

Future prospects for people with diabetes

As diabetes is a common condition and seems to be increasing in incidence world wide, there is a great deal of research into prevention, cures and treatment of any complications.

PREVENTION

The ideal treatment would be to prevent diabetes occurring at all. Our understanding of the causes of diabetes has increased dramatically over the last few decades but there is still much to be learnt. In particular we do not understand what it is that triggers the damage to the small beta (β) cells that produce insulin in the pancreas. The genes that predispose patients to this damage are being identified but precisely what they control and how the damage is initiated remain unclear. Nevertheless, once these questions are answered it is perhaps feasible that repairing these genes in patients at risk of diabetes

could prevent them developing the condition. Such a development is, however, many years away.

For type 2 diabetes, control of body weight and regular exercise are already known to reduce the chances of developing the condition. Our understanding of the genes in this type of diabetes is much less complete and full prevention is I think a distant possibility.

CURES

Many patients ask if it is not possible to have a transplant to cure their diabetes. For patients with type 1 this is an attractive prospect. If it were possible to isolate the small beta cells that make insulin and then either inject them or replace them in the patient, then insulin production should be restored. There has been a great deal of research in this area over the last few decades, but a major problem remains with rejection of the transplanted cells. In addition, actually collecting the cells from the pancreas of donors is extremely laborious and time-consuming and there would never be enough of these cells to supply all the people with diabetes world wide.

New approaches to try to take cells from either animals or from small segments of the skin of patients with diabetes, and transform them into insulin-producing cells, are exciting a great deal of interest. Many problems remain with these ideas, however, although it is possible that trials may start within the next five to ten years.

For people with type 2, the problem is more complicated because they may be making insulin but be resistant to its action. New tablets such as the thiazolidinediones were an attempt to improve insulin sensitivity but the first medicine, troglitazone, has temporarily been withdrawn because of side effects. It is very likely, however, that newer ways of altering insulin sensitivity will be developed in the not too distant future.

Insulin itself has been chemically altered to change the rate at which it is absorbed from under the skin. This has led to the development of quicker-acting and longer-acting types and some of these new 'analogues' are already available on prescription. This will provide greater flexibility for patients, particularly those with more irregular meal times.

TREATMENTS

For the vast majority of patients it is important to discover new treatments to prevent or reduce the risk of developing some of the more serious complications.

These treatments will concentrate on some of the basic mechanisms that cause eye, kidney and nerve damage. As mentioned in the chapter on complications, it seems that the exposure of these delicate structures to high glucose values for a prolonged period of time causes chemical change leading to retinopathy, nephropathy and neuropathy. Chemicals have been developed to interfere in this process in subtle ways and it may be that long-term treatment with these medicines will prevent complications. Clinical trials are both ongoing and in the early stages of planning.

Careful control of blood pressure and cholesterol levels have also been shown to be effective and it is likely that newer treatments in these areas will be developed in the next few years.

It is important to remember, however, that much can be done to reduce the risks of problems from your diabetes by regular care by both yourself and your diabetes care team. Structured supervision and examination of your eyes, urine tests, blood pressure, feet and tests for cholesterol can indicate areas for treatment which can prevent complications. Already the range of treatments and understanding of the disease has greatly improved the outlook for patients with diabetes and I am sure that this progress will be continued in the future.

KEY POINTS

✓ Prevention of diabetes remains distant for type 1, but careful diet, regular exercise and weight control reduce the chances of developing type 2

✓ Cure of insulin deficiency by transplanting or modifying cells to make insulin is the subject of intensive research

✓ New treatments to prevent or reverse complications are being developed and tested currently

Useful addresses

British Diabetic Association (BDA)
10 Queen Anne Street
London W1M 0BD
Telephone: 020 7323 1531
Fax: 020 7637 3644
Email: bda@diabetes.org.uk
Website: www.diabetes.org.uk
Useful link: www.diabetes.org.uk/bda.htm

All those suffering from diabetes are urged to join the association and thus strengthen its efforts on behalf of the diabetic community. Subscription rates are available on application to the Customer Service Department. The BDA is happy to answer any questions you may have about diabetes and offers valuable advice to members and non-members alike. Members receive *Balance*, the association's magazine, free, six times a year.

Medic-Alert Foundation
1 Bridge Wharf
156 Caledonian Road
London N1 9BR
Telephone: 020 7833 3034
Freephone: 0800 581420
Fax: 020 7278 0647
Email: info@medicalert.co.uk
Website: www.medicalert.co.uk

All people with diabetes taking insulin should join Medic-Alert. It is a charity from which identity jewellery, showing the wearer has a medical condition, may be purchased. A central file on each member is kept at headquarters and urgent medical information may be obtained by the member's doctor in an emergency. This information can be obtained on making a reverse charge telephone call from anywhere in the world. The telephone is staffed day and night.

SOS Talisman
21 Gray's Corner
Ley Street
Ilford IG2 7RQ
Tel: 020 8554 5579
Fax: 020 8554 1090
Email: sostalisman@btinternet.com

A company from which a range of identity jewellery may be purchased. Medical details are supplied on folded pieces of paper which are incorporated inside the various items of jewellery.

Index

abdomen, injecting into **27, 28**
abroad, travelling **44–5**
acarbose **22**
acromegaly and diabetes **6**
age and diabetes **4**
age-related diabetes *see* type 2 diabetes
albuminuria **58**
alcohol
– abuse and diabetes **6, 38**
– flushing following **21**
– recommendations **17–18, 38**
animal insulins **23, 41**
arterial problems **60**
athlete's foot **62**
autonomic nerves, problems **59**

baby, diabetes and **46–8**
beef insulin **23**
beta cells in pancreas **71**
– transplants **71–2**
biguanides **21–2**
bleeding after injections **28**
blindness **70**
blood pressure, raised **58, 72**
blood supply, poor **60, 61**
blood tests **7, 30–2**
– children **51**
– early morning **39**
– hospital **34–5**
– results **34**
– *see also* glucose
blurring of vision **56**
breakfasts **13**
British Diabetic Association **74**
buttocks, injecting into **27, 28**

calluses **62, 63**
carbohydrates **15–16**
– snacks **38, 43**
– for children **51, 52**
care for people with diabetes **65–7**
cataracts **56–7**

charter for people with diabetes **65–7**
children with diabetes **50–3**
chiropody **63**
chlorpropamide **21**
cholesterol levels **72**
clinics for diabetes **7**
coma
– hypoglycaemic **38–9**
– ketoacidotic **4**
complications **54–64**
corns **62, 63**
counselling for problems with children **53**
Coxsackie virus and diabetes **5**
curing diabetes **71–2**
Cushing's syndrome and diabetes **6**
cystitis **3**

definitions
– diabetes **1, 2–3**
– hormone **2–3**
dehydration **3**
delivery of baby **48**
diabetic retinopathy **57**
– diagnosis **7**
– treatment **57–8**
diagnosis of diabetes **7–9**
dialysis **58**
diet
– balanced **15–19**
– diabetes and **5–6**
– for losing weight **12, 14–15**
– treatment for diabetes **10–19**
– *see also* meals
driving and diabetes **68–9**

E111 form **33**
early warning system for hypos **39–40**
employment **69**
environmental role in diabetes **5–6**
epileptic fit from hypoglycaemia **38**
European Union, travelling to **44**

exercise **42–3, 52**
eye
– complications **56, 72**
– examination in diabetes **7**

face flushing **21**
family problems with diabetic child **52–3**
fats **16**
– breakdown **4**
feet
– problems **60–3**
– care **62**
fibre **16–17**
finger-pricking **32**
fissures in skin of feet **63**
flying **44–5**
folic acid supplements **47**
fructosamine test **35**
fruit **14**

gender and diabetes **4**
genetic role in diabetes **5, 71**
gestational diabetes **48**
glibenclamide **21**
gliclazide **21**
glipizide **21**
gliquidone **21**
glucagon
– for children **51**
– injection **39**
glucose levels
– checking **30–5, 39**
– in children **51**
– complications and **54**
– during day **24, 25**
– following meals **3**
– in pregnancy **47–8**
– in urine **33**
glucose overload in blood **2**
glucose reduction by insulin **3**
glucose storage **3**
glucose tolerance test **8**
glucose use **3**
glycated haemoglobin test **34**
glycogen storage in liver **3**

haemoglobin test, glycated **34**
height for weight chart **11**
heredity and diabetes **5, 69–70**
history of diabetes **1–2**
holidays **44–5**
hormonal diseases and diabetes **6**
hormone, definition **2–3**
human insulin **23**
hyperglycaemia **41**
hypoglycaemia **30, 36–41**
– awareness **39–41**
– causes **38**
– in children **50, 51, 52**
– definition **36**
– following tablets **20**
– night-time **39**
– preventing **36–8, 41**

– severe **38–9**
– symptoms **37**
– treating **38**
hypos see hypoglycaemia
Hypostop **39**

IDDM see type 1 diabetes
identification cards/bracelets **45**
illness and diabetes **46**
immunisation for travel **44**
impaired glucose tolerance **8**
impotence and diabetes **59**
infection, role in diabetes **5**
injection pens **25–7**
injections see insulin injections
insulin **22–9**
– analogues **72**
– deficiency **2–3**
– discovery **1–2**
– dosage during pregnancy **47–8**
– levels during day **24, 25**
– production **1–2**
– reduction of blood glucose by **3**
– resistance **3**
– storage **45**
– types **23, 41, 72**
insulin injections **10, 22–3**
– children **50**
– method **27**
– pain **28**
– reasons for **22–3**
– sites for **23, 25–8**
– timing **23–5**
– when flying **44–5**
insulin-dependent diabetes mellitus see
type 1 diabetes
insurance
– for driving **69**
– for travel **44**
islets of Langerhans **2**

jobs, diabetes and **69**

ketoacidotic coma **4**
ketones, production **4**
kidney
– problems **58, 70, 72**
– transplant **58**

lancets for finger-pricking **32**
laser treatment for retinopathy **57–8**
lipohypertrophy **27**
liver
– disease, metformin and **21**
– role in glucose use **3**
lunches/dinner **13**

malaria tablets **44**
maturity-onset diabetes see type 2
diabetes
meals
– children and **51–2, 53**
– glucose levels following **3**

– healthy eating **13, 14**
– planning to prevent hypos **37, 38, 43–4**
– regular **12**
– see also diet
Medic-Alert **46, 74**
medication for diabetes **20–9**
– adjusting before eating out **43–4**
– adjusting before exercise **42–3**
– adjusting following tests **34**
Medisense meters **32**
metformin **21–2**
microalbuminuria **58**
minerals **18–19**
monounsaturated fats **16**
motor nerves, problems **59**
mumps and diabetes **5**
muscle
– breakdown **4**
– injecting into **27**

needles **25, 28**
nerves, affected by diabetes **58–9, 72**
neuropathy **59**
– feet **61–2**
NIDDM see type 2 diabetes
night-time hypos **39**
non-insulin-dependent diabetes mellitus see type 2 diabetes

oral glucose tolerance test **8**
overweight, diabetes and **5**

pain on injections **28**
pancreas
– beta cells **71**
– insulin production in **1–2**
– where it is **2**
pancreatitis and diabetes **6**
parties, adjusting medication and food **43–4**
pens, injection **25**
pig insulin **23**
podiatry **63**
polyunsaturated fats **16**
polyuria **3**
pregnancy and diabetes **46–8**
prevention of diabetes **71**
proteins **17–18**
– breakdown **4**
– in foods **14**

retinopathy, diabetic **7, 57–8**

salads **14**
salt **18**
saturated fats **16**
SBGM **30**
secondary diabetes **6**
self blood glucose monitoring **30**
sensory nerves, problems **59**
sexual potency and diabetes **59, 69**

shoes, well-fitting **60**
signs of diabetes **3**
skin
– dryness on feet **62–3**
– injecting insulin into **23, 27**
– problems **59–60**
smoking and diabetic complications **55–5, 60**
snacks **13, 43**
SOS Talisman **74**
sports **43**
starchy carbohydrates **15–16**
starchy foods **14**
stick tests for urine **33**
stress and diabetes **6**
strips for testing blood glucose **31**
sugary carbohydrates **15**
sulphonylureas **20–1**
suppers **13**
surgical spirit for feet **62**
symptoms of diabetes **3–4**
syringes **25**

tablet treatment **20–2**
– flying and **45**
tests see blood or urine tests
thiazolidinediones **21, 72**
thighs, injecting into **27, 28**
thirst **3**
thrush **3**
toe nails **62, 63**
tolazamide **21**
tolbutamide **21**
travel **44–5, 52**
travel sickness remedies **45–6**
treatment
– by diet **10–19**
– by medication **20–9, 72–3**
troglitazone **21, 72**
twins and diabetes **5**
type 1 diabetes
– description **2**
– diagnosis **7**
– heredity **5**
– illness and **46**
– infection and **5**
– medication (insulin) **22–9**
– symptoms **4**
– transplants in **71–2**
type 2 diabetes
– description **2**
– diagnosis **7**
– environmental factors **5–6**
– heredity **5**
– illness and **46**
– prevention **71**
– symptoms **4**
– treatment **20–2**
types
– of diabetes **2**
– of insulin **23**

unsaturated fats **16**
urine
– albumin in **58**
– glucose in **3**
– passing more **3**
– tests **7, 32–4**
  – results **34**

vegetables **14**

viral infection and diabetes **5**
vitamins **18–19**

warning signs for hypos **39–40**
weight chart **11**
weight
– dieting to lose **12, 14–15**
– loss and diagnosing diabetes **3**